Intermittent Fasting for Women:

The Easy and Complete Guide for Weight Loss, Control Hunger, Burn fats in Healthy and Simple ways

Table of Contents

Introduction

Congratulations on downloading *Intermittent Fasting for Women* and taking the first step on the path to a happier, stronger you through fasting.

Dieting is complicated, especially as a woman. With so much information and so many products and programs on the market, it's difficult to know which one will work for you. As women, there are also many physical and psychological factors that affect how the body absorbs, stores, and processes calories consumed throughout the day. All of this can negatively affect weight improvement in women, and it can be easy to get discouraged when progress is slow despite your best effort.

Using this guide, you will gain an unquestionable understanding of Intermittent Fasting, how it can be effective for weight loss, and how it works specifically with the female form. With this, you can decide if fasting is right for you, and if so, how to choose the right schedule. You will also learn about how choosing the best foods and diet plan when fasting will maximize your overall advancement.

The Intermittent Fasting for Women will provide you with the tools you need to get started including:

- Everything you could ever want to know about Intermittent Fasting, the science behind it, and how it works with the female body.
- How to determine your body type and why this is important to know when starting any kind of diet or fitness program.
- Diet recommendations with detailed information on the programs and recipes to try.
- A rundown of the most widely practiced Intermittent Fasting techniques and exercises.
- A 14-Day Beginner's Guide with step-by-step instructions on beginning your fasting schedule.

Thank you for downloading *Intermittent Fasting for Women*. Remember that fasting is an easy and adaptable way to improve your overall health and wellness whether your goal is weight loss or simply enhancing your lifestyle. Best wishes as you work toward your health goals and enjoy the guide!

Chapter 1: Getting to Know Intermittent Fasting

Fasting is performed across the globe for a variety of personal reasons. From being applied as a form of religious devotion to being employed to improve one's health and lifestyle, fasting is a widely respected practice with centuries of evidence to support its effectiveness and benefits. With all the research and scientific support available, there are still people who question it as a health tool. It's understandable considering all the time spent in high school health classes being taught the importance of not skipping meals.

In most cases, this hesitation comes from not having the right information about fasting and how it is being utilized as a helpful weight loss option. The goal of this guide is to help you expand your knowledge and feel more comfortable with the concept of Intermittent Fasting so you can take advantage of all the benefits the program has to offer.

What Is Intermittent Fasting?

Fasting is the process of decreasing your overall calorie intake by markedly restricting or eliminating your food consumption for a determined period of time. Intermittent Fasting is a dieting system designed around the basic practice of fasting but on a consistent and long-term basis. Intermittent Fasting can be used to reach short-term weight loss goals, but it is most effective for those looking to make a lifestyle change.

Often described as a dieting pattern, Intermittent Fasting gives each person has the freedom to choose how and when he or she wants to fast to get the most out of their fasting periods. One way you have control with the program is determining how you are going to fast. A common misunderstanding people have about fasting is that you're only doing it right if you're starving yourself. While completely avoiding food consumption is one way to fast, the more commonly practiced method where health and weight loss are concerned involves simply reducing your calorie intake during fasting times. The standard recommendation for food reduction fasting is to limit your calorie allowance to a quarter of your typical daily intake.

Not everyone who tries fasting is physically able to avoid eating entirely. Sometimes this is due to existing dietary health issues that could be negatively affected by a change in eating habits. Others, usually those new to fasting and dieting, don't have the willpower or physical stamina for this when they first start. The beauty of Intermittent Fasting is that your body never reaches the point of starvation. You choose and adopt a fasting schedule to fit your individual needs so there is never a period where you fast long enough that your body suffers from a lack of nutrients.

At its very core, Intermittent Fasting is something all humans already do while we sleep. For most, adapting to their chosen program simply involves prolonging this period of time where we aren't eating or consuming any high-calorie liquids.

Fasting Through the Ages: The Origins of Intermittent Fasting

Fasting has been practiced in one form or another since the beginning of mankind. The first recorded use of fasting as a health treatment dates back to ancient Greece and the patriarch of practiced medicine, Hippocrates of Kos. Hippocrates is most known for laying the foundation for medical procedures and practices that are still in use today. He is even the inspiration behind the Hippocratic Oath, a pledge all medical professionals must make to uphold unquestionable ethical standards when caring for patients.

One of his most commonly assigned treatments for illness, especially affecting the stomach or digestive tract, was to avoid food for a certain amount of time, ingesting only apple cider vinegar until the symptoms cleared. The thinking behind this was to allow the body to fight the illness and recover on its own without having to worry about further ingesting something harmful that may have been the initial source of the sickness. By not eating, the patients also gave their body the time it needed to process and expel the sickness without further fueling it with calories and chemicals broken down in digestion.

Medicine in ancient times was inspired by observing nature. When humans and other animals are feeling ill, it is in our nature not to eat. Instinctually, the body knows that ingesting food when fighting sickness or discomfort only makes it more difficult to beat the symptoms and get back on your feet. That is why most people turn to light options, such as chicken noodle soup, when they have a cold or find themselves dealing with stomach troubles.

As time progressed, fasting remained a constant topic of conversation in medical circles. For those who are new to or have never taken much interest in treatment techniques, fasting is usually associated with a religious ceremony. Nearly all existing religions, particularly those with the most ancient roots, incorporate a form of fasting into their beliefs.

Buddhism promotes a form of Intermittent Fasting where practitioners only eat in the early morning hours and then fast from noon to the early hours of the next day. In this case, fasting for their physical and spiritual wellbeing is an ordinary part of their daily lives. In Islamic practice, Muslims only fast throughout their holy month of Ramadan. During this time, as proof of their devotion to their beliefs, they fast absolutely (even eliminating their water and liquid consumption) from the time the sun rises until it sets in the evening. The rest of the year, Muslims are free to eat normally within the dietary restrictions of their religion.

Due to the risk of dehydration and an issue with increased calorie consumption during the nighttime hours, this form of fasting is not recommended for those using it as a means of improving their overall strength and wellness.

In the modern health world, there are several different medical professionals credited with refining and popularizing different Intermittent Fasting methods (which we will talk more about later when we break down the techniques).

Why Are So Many People Embracing Intermittent Fasting?

Despite deeply programmed ideas against going longer periods of time without eating, more and more people are turning to Intermittent Fasting when they are ready to make a change that enhances their physical health, supports a longer life, and ensures they can be active for every moment of it.

Convenient & Adaptable

In addition to the many health benefits of Intermittent Fasting, people appreciate the convenient nature of the program and the freedom to fit their fasting schedule into their established daily lives. There are no complicated routines to follow, no specialty foods or vitamins to order, and no expensive equipment to sit and collect dust in the living room corner. It simply comes down to understanding the different Intermittent Fasting methods and choosing the one that works for you.

If you start an Intermittent Fasting routine and discover that the technique you chose or the schedule you set for your fasting times isn't working for you, then you can alter the program to meet your needs. For example, you have a fasting schedule where you eat normally for two days and then completely fast for 24 hours before returning to your regular eating habits. You have given your body some time to adjust but are still having issues with painful hunger during fasting times or intolerable fatigue throughout the day.

One way to remedy these issues without abandoning Intermittent Fasting as a dietary option is to limit your calorie consumption to 25% of your average daily level during fasting times instead of avoiding food entirely. Another option would be to try a different technique that guides you through fasting for a number of hours each day instead of for a full 24-hour period.

Intermittent Fasting: The Chosen Method of the Stars

When it comes to gaining popularity, celebrity endorsements never hurt. Even Hollywood has embraced Intermittent Fasting as a meaningful diet that strengthens the mind while training the body. Celebrities such as Hugh Jackman, known for his iconic role as Wolverine in Marvel's *X-Men* films and Chris Pratt of the *Jurassic World* movies both swear by fasting as a method for not only losing weight but for building muscle. Actress Kate Walsh from TV's *Private Practice* received orders from her doctor to fast in order to avoid storing excess water weight and heightening mental clarity.

Social media is buzzing with posts and tweets from celebrities about how much progress they have made toward their health goals simply by controlling when they allow themselves to eat.

Extend Your Life & Enjoy the Extra Time

Another factor bringing people into the world of Intermittent Fasting is the science supporting how fasting can help the body fight the aging process. Over time, fasting changes the body on a cellular level; altering the way the cells in our body react to the consumption of calories, (we'll cover this in more detail in the next chapter).

The cells become stronger without the constant presence of calories in the body and are better able to resist the aging hormones and combat the natural process of degeneration over time. The body adapts to the caloric restriction and learns to burn energy more efficiently; paying more attention to getting consumed nutrients to where they are most needed for daily function. Muscles become stronger, internal organs improve performance, and mental processes intensify and learn to be resilient as the body reaches higher levels of health consciousness.

The Golden Rules of Intermittent Fasting

Although it is embraced for its convenience and simplicity, there are certain base rules all Intermittent Fasting programs should follow in order to make sure you are getting the most out of your fasting routine.

#1: Choose the Time of Day That Works Best for You

With so many different ways to benefit from fasting, there is no pressure for you to stick to one way just because that's how you've seen or read about other people doing it.

Start by thinking about your schedule and asking yourself:

- What time do you wake up?
- How late are you up at night?

- When are you at your most active?
- When do you work out?

These are all good questions to ask yourself before you start any Intermittent Fasting routine. When you need to eat is determined by when your body needs the most energy to operate smoothly. Most people will tell you they prefer to skip breakfast and eat later in the day when fasting on a daily schedule. However, those who wake up later in the mornings and are most active into the later hours of the evening tend to benefit from eating earlier in their day, so they have the energy to make it through their active evenings without having to break their fasting period.

The fundamental component of determining the effectiveness of Intermittent Fasting, regardless of technique or schedule, is consistency and discipline. It's not a matter of fasting when everyone else is fasting just because that timeframe works for them. It's a matter of sticking to it and not surrendering when outside forces try to distract you from your goals.

#2: Don't Let Your Coffee Set You Back

Since there will be fewer or no spare calories to draw energy from, it is critical to maintain the body's hydration levels during periods of fasting. Even though food ingestion will be limited, nearly all forms of fasting allow you to consume any fluids that are free from or have few calories per serving.

Those looking to see more rapid results stay hydrated with water alone. Water contains no calories and is more often than not, readily available no matter where the day may take you. It is also something that people have access to in their homes, meaning that there is no need to spend money on unnecessary low-calorie drinks.

For those who find it difficult to only drink water or cannot function without their morning dose of caffeine, coffee and tea are allowed for consumption during fasting periods. One issue most people don't even realize they're facing with drinking tea and coffee is the temptation for mixing in additional ingredients that add unexpected calories to their fasting drinks. There are many people who can't drink coffee without milk or creamer and those who cannot drink tea or coffee without sugar. If you are choosing to drink more than water during fasting periods, make sure that you are a careful about controlling your liquid calorie intake, especially in the early days of fasting when it is most likely to slip your mind.

If you do find yourself needing a low-calorie boost that won't counteract your fasting, try this green juice recipe. It is rich in vitamins and nutrients that will support your brain function and internal systems without filling your body with the calories you are working so hard to avoid. This juice is particularly useful before working out and during the day when weariness starts to affect your work or performance. The ingredients are easy to find at your local supermarket and fit with almost any program you may be following, including vegan and gluten-free diets.

If you don't have a juicer, this recipe also works as a smoothie simply by adding ice and combining in a blender until smooth.

Glorious Green Juice/Smoothie

Prep Time: 5 to 10 minutes

Total Time: 10-15 minutes

Makes 1 serving

Ingredients

1 large apple

2 medium-to-large oranges

1 small lime

3 cups fresh spinach, washed and patted dry

½ cup fresh parsley, shredded

1 tablespoon powdered ginger root

*If making a smoothie, also include 1 cup of fresh water and 1 to 2 cups of ice depending on texture and portion preferences

Directions for Juice

- Combine all ingredients in a juicer and blend until smooth. Pour over ice or store in the refrigerator until thoroughly chilled.

For Smoothies

- Add ice and water to blender.

- Chop the apple, spinach, and fresh parsley into small to medium bits to ensure they blend entirely into the drink.
- Halve the oranges and lime, and then remove the seeds from inside. Squeeze each one of them over the blender, collecting the juice and any pulp that comes loose.
- Add the powdered ginger root and blend until smooth.
- As you blend, add more ice for a thicker texture or more water if it needs thinning out.

Feel free to add any powdered vitamins or supplements you may take to the juice or smoothie. Additional spices can be added for flavor as well. Just be careful that you do not add any ingredients that will increase the calorie count.

#3: Understand the Connection Between Fitness & Fasting

We have already started talking about the importance of timing when it comes to being able to function during fasting periods. Like with any diet or weight loss program, you will see your best results by bolstering your fasting regiment with regular exercise.

However, when you initially begin an Intermittent Fasting routine, it is important to consider that your body will need time to adjust to running on a reduced calorie consumption. This is particularly good to take into account for first-time fasters and those who start their fasting schedule in the middle of their busy week as it can become complicated to tell whether any discomfort you may feel is the body adjusting to the fasting or reacting to environmental stresses. For these reasons, most Intermittent Fasting supporters agree that during fasting periods, you should only work out if you have the energy to do so.

You can give yourself some energy by consuming a small number of calories from fruit and vegetable-based drinks, such as the green juice mentioned above. This helps provide some balance in the body between the calories consumed before a workout and the calories burned through exercise so that you essentially break even instead of overextending your stored energy. If you find that you can only work out during fasting periods, this is one way to avoid physical and mental exhaustion which can lead to frustration and lack of willpower.

The best way to keep from straining yourself when adjusting to and maintaining a fasting schedule is to plan your workouts so that you are exercising just after you've eaten. You can do this by working out during the hours in which you are free to eat, but you can also do this by planning your exercises at the beginning of your fasting periods. This gives your body time to rest and recover while you fast.

#4: Stay Moving & Stay Motivated

While you may not have the energy for a full body workout, it is helpful to keep yourself active when you're awake and fasting. The reason for this is because most of us turn to mindless snacking or daydreaming about food when we're bored and know we shouldn't be eating. If you find temptation flooding your mind when you're fasting, find some way to distract yourself and keep your will strong.

Some ways to keep these thoughts from controlling you and stay on schedule with your fasting include:

- **Taking a walk outside**: It doesn't have to be long or fast-paced. Often times, a leisurely stroll in the fresh air is enough to revitalize the mind and body, no matter what physical or emotional trials you may be facing. Go to the local park or just around the block a few times. Just get up and get moving!

- **Saving your chores for downtime:** This won't work with everyone's schedules, but one way to conquer your cravings while fasting is to use any downtime you have to focus on household tasks. Maybe there is some laundry you have been meaning to fold or a closet full of old boxes you want to sort through. These may seem like trivial distractions, but they are the perfect escapes from tempting or disheartening thoughts.

- **Picking up a Hobby:** As adults, many of us don't have any time to even think about having a hobby. We become overwhelmed by deadlines and obligations that any free time we usually have is spent scrolling through social media or in front of the TV. However, if you find yourself struggling with the urge to snack while you fast, then it may be the perfect time dust off that book you've been meaning to read or finish that puzzle that's been sitting on the shelf since you brought it home a few years back.

- **Getting out of the house:** Call up some friends, go for a drive. Temptation strikes when we're at our most comfortable and our most vulnerable, so basically whenever we are home with nothing to occupy our time. You will run into distractions and impulses whenever you are out in society, but there is also so much more to keep you active and away from negative influences.

Many of us eat as a compulsive habit, instead of as a necessity. It's something that we do unconsciously, taking comfort from the food and the repetitive plate to face movements. This is one of the first things people notice and struggle with when they start Intermittent Fasting. Everyone has their own way to combat it. Don't hesitate to try new things and explore while you search for yours!

#5: Consistency is Key

Maintaining a healthy lifestyle is hard, particularly if you are adapting to major changes from a lifetime of unhealthy eating and behavior. There will be times when you falter and times when you fail. There will times where you cave to temptation or abandon your fasting schedule on a particularly difficult day. It is natural to get frustrated and dampened when these challenges arise, but never forget that you can always bounce back and get back on track.

If you let doubt and other negative thoughts cloud your mind, it becomes easier and easier to reject your weight loss plan and retreat to the emotional security of old habits. It is these times of trial that we can be our own worst enemies. Never forget that you may not be able to control everything that happens around you, but you are always in control of how you react to it.

While you always want to give it your best effort, it is okay if you fumble from time to time. It is important to accept that this will happen before you commit to an Intermittent Fasting program or you are setting yourself up for failure. What matters is how you recover from these moments of vulnerability. Do you get disheartened and quit? Or do you shake it off and start fresh with your fasting tomorrow? All failure is in the past now. Focus your energy on maintaining that forward momentum!

Chapter 2: The Skinny on Intermittent Fasting & Women

There are a lot of contradicting opinions regarding whether women should take part in fasting for weight loss or its other health benefits. The main reason for this is that in studies done over the last century; women's bodies have reacted differently to fasting than men who fasted for the same hours, over the same length of time. With so much information and promotion out there, it can be difficult to decide whether Intermittent Fasting is right for you. In this chapter, we will cover not only the positive aspects of Intermittent Fasting but also potential risks and difficulties that others have reported regarding their fasting experience.

Does this mean that women should not avoid fasting? Absolutely not. Women just face different challenges with fasting which means that every woman will have unique modifications they make to their Intermittent Fasting schedule. It's recommended by fitness professionals, nutritionists, and medical experts alike that women take a more relaxed attitude when it comes to fasting than men do, so they can prevent any damaging changes or complications to vital, female-specific body functions.

The female body relies on calorie intake and hormone balances more than males do, and both are major factors affected once fasting begins. What women should remember when researching and planning their Intermittent Fasting schedule is that it is better to start by lowering calorie intake as a form of fasting for shorter periods of time as opposed to jumping into full fasting mode on alternate days. Once the body adjusts to the change, then calorie intake can be decreased again or time fasting can be increased until you reach the level you're striving for.

The Advantages & Benefits of Intermittent Fasting

Anyone who keeps their ears perked for updates on the latest health trends has heard about the benefits of Intermittent Fasting and why everyone is loving it. There are countless reviews and blog posts circulating the internet about personal modifications that made the program effective for individuals and the fasting success stories that follow. People of all ages are praising Intermittent Fasting for their advanced health and wellness level and can't wait to inspire as many as they can with progress photos and helpful tips.

Some of the advantages of choosing Intermittent Fasting as your preferred method of weight loss include:

- <u>Convenience:</u> Making time and effort with daily dieting and exercising can be difficult enough that adding a fasting schedule into the mix sounds agonizing! One of the reasons people are embracing Intermittent Fasting is that you don't have to conform to a strict routine. You have the power to set your fasting times around your existing schedule, meaning that you can fast when it works best for you.

- Simplicity: Intermittent Fasting is straightforward and easy to master once you've done the proper research and have a firm understanding of it. Once you have chosen your schedule and the best times to promote your fasting success, all you have to do is get started. There are no subscriptions or gym memberships. No expensive equipment, ingredients, or supplements to buy. Most people on Intermittent Fasting plans actually find themselves saving money over time as they buy less food for their non-fasting breaks as their body adjusts to reduced daily calorie intake.

- Works with Any Diet: Since the Intermittent Fasting system does not tell you what to eat, you never have to worry about adjusting your diet if you already have one that you're happy and seeing success with. Anyone looking to change what they eat when they start fasting should focus on low calorie, high protein diets that will serve to enhance the weight loss and health benefits that come with Intermittent Fasting.

More good news for those ready to start their own Intermittent Fasting schedule is that there are as many health benefits as there are advantages to the program!

One major benefit of Intermittent Fasting that dates back to the early days of medicine states that it detoxifies and cleanses the body of harmful elements and energies. Once these toxins are expelled, the body has the opportunity to heal muscle and cellular deterioration, stabilize digestive health, and help the brain regulate sleeping patterns.

There are a variety of other physical benefits Intermittent Fasting participants enjoy including:

- Heightened mental clarity and brain function
- Triggering autophagy (the process of replacing degraded parts of a cell with fresh cellular material) in the body and the start of cellular cleansing
- Improved overall fat burning through digestion
- Lower cholesterol and blood sugar levels
- Decrease in inflammation throughout the body
- The potential to increase total life span and promote physical ability during the later years

Some people also see an increase in muscle mass as they lose weight. While this is more common in males, females also benefit from the weight loss and muscle building aspects of regular Intermittent Fasting.

One of the most astonishing benefits reported by people struggling with diabetic symptoms or other blood sugar related diseases is that Intermittent Fasting has helped them improve their vital numbers. Along with their professionally prescribed medicine, fasters have seen notable differences in their body's resistance to insulin leading to a lower chance of developing Type 2 diabetes. In some cases, fasters have even seen a reversal in their existing diabetic symptoms with the balance of Intermittent Fasting, medical treatment, exercise, and proper dieting.

Another benefit of those utilizing the Intermittent Fasting program love is that weight loss while fasting comes from all parts of the body, including the core or belly area. The core is where most people, especially women, tend to store the majority of their body fat. Intermittent Fasting targets the larger fat stores in the body. This means that those who struggle with losing weight and mass in this area specifically should start to see some reduction once their body has adapted to fasting.

This chart shows the results of a three-week study on first-time Intermittent Fasting participants. The study volunteers whose measurements were taken and the individual's progress can be seen below.

Total Measurement Change (in inches)		
Body Part	**Start**	**Week 3**
Bicep	13	12.5
Chest	37.5	36.5
Waist	33	31
Neck	12	12
Thigh	24.5	24
Calf	16	15.5
Hip	42	40
Total Inches Lost		**6.5 inches**

Things to Consider Before You Try Intermittent Fasting

Yes, it's exciting to think about starting a fasting schedule when you read about the benefits or see your friends and favorite stars posting about how well Intermittent Fasting has worked for them. However, Intermittent Fasting is a serious commitment for both your mind and body that requires dedication and perseverance. Intermittent Fasting, if not done properly, can also have lasting negative effects on the body which can be counteracted if you know what to watch for.

The majority of these side effects fade when the body adjusts to the calorie changes with time, once fasting has become a habit or once a fasting routine has been abandoned (depending on if you are just starting or coming to the end of an Intermittent Fasting plan). Despite their temporary nature, any negative reactions your body displays when you start fasting should not be ignored and should be discussed with your personal physician if they become severe.

One issue many people don't consider before fasting is that it is more effective, and you are more likely to continue with your Intermittent Fasting regiment if you let yourself ease into it in steps. This is particularly important for first-time fasters. Your goal may be to fast for 18 to 24-hour periods on alternating days, but that can be a major shock to the body and can lead to physical discomfort and mental exhaustion. If you've never fasted before or haven't fasted for a long time, it is better to start with a milder fasting plan, so your body has time to adjust and prepare for each next step. The more time you give your body to adapt, the fewer potential negative effects you'll see as you continue to fast.

Social media has provided people with an outlet to share and document everything they do in their daily lives. This deeply ingrained need to show ourselves off means that most people are already used to taking pictures of themselves and their activities to post to their friends. One thing most people who have made great strides in their weight loss and health improvement will tell you is they wish or are glad they had taken progress pictures each step of the way. Even if you have no intention of sharing them with anyone else, progress pictures are a great motivational tool to rejuvenate your faith in and reignite your dedication to your Intermittent Fasting schedule. There will be difficult days and temptation is always just around the corner. The more tools you have to draw strength from, the better your chances are of not caving or quitting.

Remember, there's no such thing as knowing too much about a topic so don't skimp on your research. This is especially important if you have read the blog posts and talked to people who already do Intermittent Fasting and still have doubts or concerns about your own health opportunities with fasting.

Our Foundations & the Pre-Historic Predicament

One issue women face is that in some cases, women who stop fasting see a slight weight gain in the days that follow as their overall food intake increases and their diet normalizes. This is a natural defensive response to a sudden increase in calorie consumption that the female body has developed through time and which dates back to the early days of humanity. Early humans were hunters and gatherers who relied solely on their environment for food. Without any means of refrigeration or preservation, they would only hunt for what they needed and never knew where their next meal was coming from. They would experience periods of fasting when food scarce where their bodies had to learn to run on fewer calories. Needing calories to function and not knowing when more would come, the human body adapted to storing the majority of calories consumed and storing them in the fat cells to create a physical effect we now know as "water weight."

Genetics researchers believe that it's during this time period that the body made the evolutionary changes in genetics and hormones seen in modern humans. This is why women see a slight weight gain in the first few days following a long period of Intermittent Fasting. Having adjusted to fluctuating food consumption, women's bodies take full advantage of the extra calories they receive once they stop fasting; storing them to pull from the next time they need some extra energy. It's an instinctual, unconscious response that roots into our very nature as human beings.

Not all women experience this initial increase in weight, but for those that do, there are ways to combat it. The good news about water weight is that once the body adjusts to the increased caloric intake that weight will drop off again.

Women who fast can also minimize or eliminate this issue by decreasing their Intermittent Fasting in stages when they are ready to stop. For those completely excluding food during fasting periods, gradually end your fasting with these steps. Remember to give your body time to adjust at each stage before moving forward.

1. Decrease the amount of time you fast and avoid increasing calorie consumption by eating the same or close to the number of calories you normally consume when not fasting. For example, spread out your eating over your extra time with lower calorie meals consumed more frequently instead of one or two larger meals eaten before fasting again.

2. Increase your calorie intake during fasting periods by 25% of your daily calorie consumption every two weeks. Do this until you are consuming the same number of calories on former fasting days as you were on eating days and your diet has normalized.

3. If you see an increase in your weight at any time throughout the plan, increase your exercise in small

increments until you see the water weight disappear. You can do this by slightly increasing your workout intensity, adding half an hour to your routine, going for an extra lap around the block or maybe just taking the stairs wherever you go to help burn those extra calories your body is holding on to.

Remember that these steps are just recommendations and that you can adjust your plan to fit how your body responds to caloric changes, should you ever want to stop fasting. Talk to your doctor with any questions you have about more fasting options and personalized program adjustments.

Hormones & Handling Your Health

As a woman, there are several basic, but critical roles linked to calorie consumption and the body's metabolic function. At its most primal level, the female body was developed and perfected over time for fertility and human reproduction. Fasting in women, especially those who haven't fasted before, affects the body's hormones in a way that men's bodies don't share. Here is a closer look at some of the hormones affected by Intermittent Fasting and how women can both identify and oppose any changes.

Estrogen & Progesterone

Estrogen imbalance is a serious health concern for women of all ages. It is a fundamental hormone or the female body and having balanced levels of estrogen and progesterone is imperative for conserving complete physical health as a woman. Estrogen and progesterone contribute to major bodily functions in women such as metabolic performance, cognitive function, ability to handle anxiety and stress, and general emotional stability.

Potential signs that your estrogen levels are imbalanced include:

- Lower energy levels and increased muscle fatigue
- Decreased total bone density and muscle tone
- Infertility, changes to menstruation and other reproductive issues
- Weight gain and increased blood sugar levels

For women trying to get pregnant, estrogen imbalance from reduced calorie consumption can affect the female reproductive cycle and even shrink the ovaries over time. While there are still few tests focused on human female fasting effects, there have been extensive studies performed on female rats and the way their bodies reacted to fasting periods, specifically with regards to hormone balance and reproductive functions. These studies found that in up to two weeks after fasting began, some of the female test subjects showed lower levels of estrogen, reduced fertility, and smaller ovaries while others showed little to no change.

The reason for this is that long or fluctuating periods of fasting can send the female body into a type of survival mode. This instinctual need to focus on survival tells the body to pull away from using precious calories on non-essential roles like preparing for a baby you aren't expecting and use them more constructively on maintaining vital bodily functions. This is why it is crucial for women that are planning on having a baby, within the next few years at least, to eat normally and carry on with a healthy level of calorie consumption for their body type and weight.

Another concern women should take into account when considering how fasting is affecting their hormones is that one hormonal imbalance has the potential to prompt another. In most cases where women have reported issues revolving around their estrogen levels, that imbalance has been the cause of or worsened an existing hormonal imbalance in the thyroid. The thyroid is a critical gland in the neck that is directly connected to the body's metabolic processes. Hormone imbalances in the thyroid can negatively affect the metabolism and how it behaves.

When it comes down to, hormonal health and balance with Intermittent Fasting for women is a complicated topic and how the body will react to fasting cannot be predicted. The only way to truly know how your body will react to Intermittent Fasting is to make a plan with all the knowledge you've collected and try your chosen schedule for two weeks to see what changes, if any, you notice.

Intermittent Fasting & Menopause

Menopause is a grueling time for women, and there is so much that women in the post-menopausal phase have to learn to adjust to without needing to worry about aggravating their symptoms by introducing a fasting program into their daily lives. The decreased estrogen levels throughout the body cause the fat distribution to change, making fat cells collect in new areas and in some cases, causing unexpected weight gain.

A common opinion among fitness and health professionals is that menopausal and post-menopausal women get to experience the most health and wellness benefits of Intermittent Fasting than any other gender or age group. Studies have shown that post-menopausal women especially tend to lose up to twice as much weight as anyone else on the same or similar fasting schedules.

One reason for this is that women going through or finished with menopause are statistically more likely to stick to their diets and fasting schedule than pre-menopausal women. Another reason is that women in this category are coming to the end of or through with their menstrual cycles and the body knows it no longer needs to expend calories on the reproductive systems. The risk of hormonal imbalances is also reduced post-menopause as the body adapts to lower levels of estrogen. Therefore, it becomes easier to adjust to a reduced calorie diet and a more challenging Intermittent Fasting technique.

When Women Should Not Try Intermittent Fasting

While women are encouraged to take advantage of all the benefits Intermittent Fasting has to offer, there are exceptions and certain circumstances in which women should maintain their normal calorie intake.

One of these circumstances is pregnancy. Women who are pregnant may be pregnant or are trying to get pregnant should never partake in fasting of any kind. In fact, experts and nutritionists recommend pregnant women add 300 to 500 calories to their regular diet throughout their second and third trimesters. This is also the time when pregnant women experience the most fluctuations in their vital blood readings. For example, most women report sudden drops in blood pressure and blood sugar during pregnancy, regardless of whether or not they were fasting or eating the recommended number of calories per day.

Some of the health risks of fasting while pregnant include:

- An increase in the possibility of premature birth
- Increases the potential of low birth weight for the baby
- Lack of fundamental vitamins for the mother and the child
- Higher risks of health complications for the mother both during and after pregnancy

There have also been reports theorizing that fasting during pregnancy can lead to health complications later in life for the child, but there is still not enough evidence to fully substantiate that. When it comes down to it, one of the main reasons people take up Intermittent Fasting is to lose weight, which is something women shouldn't be focused on during pregnancy.

With this knowledge in hand, it is not impossible for women to continue fasting while pregnant, but it is only considered safe for women who have already been fasting for a minimum of two years before becoming pregnant. Those who have been fasting so long that it is second nature to them and are worried about how increasing their calorie consumption could affect their body should speak with their doctor about the best way for them to move forward.

All pregnant women should stay away from refined sugars and processed foods, focusing their food consumption on proteins and good carbohydrates to ensure the body has everything it needs to preserve the health of both the mother and the baby.

Children of a certain age should also stay away from fasting. In their younger years, children need all the vitamins and nutrients they can consume to grow up fit and healthy. Children also have higher metabolisms, so it is important to make sure they receive the recommended number of calories per day they need to avoid any health complications.

Girls younger than or going through their puberty phase should not participate in fasting. This is the time in most women's lives that the risk of hormone imbalance is at its highest and has the greatest effect on the body. Fasting through puberty can lead to complications with a woman's fertility and ability to sustain proper estrogen levels throughout her life.

People who are already underweight or have had trouble with eating disorders in the past should also avoid fasting of any kind. Consciously deciding not to eat (even for shorter periods of time) can trigger negative habits and impulses psychologically connected to disorders such as anorexia and bulimia. Those who struggle with maintaining a healthy weight for their age and physical build will not benefit from Intermittent Fasting because their bodies have little to no extra weight to shed and are typically already acting in some form of survival mode. These people are also encouraged to stay away from Intermittent Fasting, so they don't increase their risk of health problems by further limiting their calorie intake.

Intermittent Fasting for Super Moms

Moms are constantly running around and taking care of others, so much so that many busy moms can forget about their personal health as they focus on the health and wellness of their family. It can be difficult to find time for exercising and become easy to cave to cravings with kitchens full of snacks for the kids.

Intermittent Fasting is becoming more and more popular with active moms looking to lose weight, increase muscle tone or improve their overall energy flow. Thanks to the simplicity and convenience, most moms find it a breeze to design their Intermittent Fasting times around their hectic schedules.

Intermittent Fasting as a mom presents its own challenges, but the more you know, the more you will be able to foresee, prepare for or adapt to (if necessary) trials as they come.

Fasting Through Motherhood Can Be Exhausting

One of the most common effects fasting moms face that others on the Intermittent Fasting program may not have to deal with is a noticeable decrease in energy. This is particularly true in the months following birth. There are other factors that play into this concern. Factors like how demanding each mom's daily schedule is, how many children she cares for, the mother's age and what kind of diet she is following when not fasting, but insufficient calorie consumption plays a powerful role in energy generation and use.

While one of the general benefits of Intermittent Fasting is an increase in energy and overall wellness, women (moms in particular) have to carefully monitor their hormonal changes, the risks of which are potentially long-lasting and various as we discussed earlier.

One modification for mothers who find themselves needing a boost of energy during their fast can do is turn to low calorie, high protein smoothies (for those avoiding food completely) or low calorie, high protein snacks (for those simply reducing calories during fasting periods).

The following recipe is a good example of the kind of juice, smoothie or other drink that provides essential vitamins the body can use for energy without undermining your Intermittent Fasting periods.

Energizing Avocado Smoothie

Prep Time: 5 to 10 minutes

Total Time: 10 to 15 minutes

Makes 1 serving

Ingredients

1 large banana

1 medium to large avocado, ripe

1 medium lime

25 to 50 fresh mint leaves, depending on your personal taste

2 cups almond milk

A handful of dark chocolate chips (to taste)

Directions

- Chop the banana and meat of the avocado into small or medium-sized chunks to ensure a smooth breakdown. Drop in a blender.
- Add mint, chocolate and almond milk to blender.
- Juice lime into mixture and add 1 to 2 cups of ice.
- Blend until smooth or preferred texture and serve immediately or allow to chill in the refrigerator until cool.

For those moms searching for a high protein snack to boost energy without having to markedly increase their calorie consumption, try these Bake-Free Oatmeal Energy Bombs!

Bake-Free Oatmeal Energy Bombs

Prep Time: 5 to 10 minutes

Total Time: 10 minutes

Makes 10 to 20 energy bombs (depending on the size of bites rolled)

Ingredients

1 cup rolled oats

½ cup preferred miniature chocolate chips (dark chocolate is recommended)

2 to 3 tablespoons ground flax seed

¼ teaspoon vanilla extract

4 tablespoon all-natural honey (organic is best)

½ cup peanut butter, preferred nut butter or peanut butter substitute (for those with allergies)

Directions

- Add all ingredients to a medium to large bowl and mix together by hand or with a spoon until combined.

- Once evenly mixed, roll handfuls of the mixture into about 1 to 1½ inch bites.
- Place bites on a plate or a tray and place in the refrigerator or freezer until fully set. This usually takes 30 to 90 minutes.

Pro Tip: If you find the mixture too sticky or difficult to handle when it is first combined, refrigerate it for 20 minutes. This will cool it and make it more suitable to roll into balls.

The energy bombs are ready to go as soon as they are set, but they will last up to a week in the refrigerator or 3 months in the freezer if kept in an airtight container.

Both of these recipes will provide you with the all the extra energy you need while satisfying your sweet tooth and guaranteeing you don't break any part of your fast.

Breastfeeding While Fasting

For new moms and moms who have just given birth, there can be some confusion and hesitation around whether or not it is safe or right to fast during the breastfeeding phase. Women committed to their Intermittent Fasting routine but also concerned for their breastfeeding child's wellbeing can rest easily. There is no scientific evidence to suggest that there is any danger in breastfeeding while fasting at normal intervals.

The body adjusts the way it typically burns calories while breastfeeding to account for milk production. This is considered one of the essential bodily functions by your brain during the breastfeeding period, ensuring that an appropriate number of all calories consumed will be dedicated to producing enough milk to keep the baby healthy.

Those who fast for longer than 24 hours at a time (usually for spiritual or religious reasons) may see a decline in milk production or early weaning from their child, but those fasting on a regular or alternating schedule for no longer than 12 to 16 hours at a time should not see any change. However, if you are fasting while breastfeeding and have any concerns about the amount or potency of the milk your body is producing then you should speak with your doctor about all potential issues and recommended solutions.

Is Intermittent Fasting the Right Choice for You?

If you don't fall into any of the high-risk categories we've covered and don't have any pre-existing medical issues related to caloric or metabolic functions, you are good to go to start your Intermittent Fasting experience.

Other thoughts to consider and questions to answer before starting any kind of fasting:

- Why do I want to start Intermittent Fasting? What is my main goal?
- How do I want to fast? Completely or with reduced calories during fasting times?
- When do I want to fast and how long will I fast for?
- What kind of diet do I want to follow when I can eat?
- What day will I start my fasting?

- Have I considered both the pros and cons of the Intermittent Fasting program?

Once you have a strong understanding of how to start, you are free to begin your Intermittent Fasting journey! It is always recommended to speak with your doctor before starting any new diet or exercise program and Intermittent Fasting is no exception.

Chapter 3: Understanding How What You Eat Affects You

Understanding how Intermittent Fasting will affect you is only one part of starting your fasting plan. In order to totally appreciate how fasting works, it is imperative to get a better understanding of how the body processes what we eat. Once you have, you will be able to choose a new diet plan or make adjustments to your current diet in order to maximize your weight loss potential with Intermittent Fasting.

What Happens to What We Eat

We all know that everything we eat goes to our stomachs where it is broken down through the process of digestion, but many people don't know or have never thought about what exactly is being broken down and what the body does with it. Our bodies rely on us to consume not only the correct amount of food to promote our personal health but also the right foods to support the physical processes that are activated when we fast.

When we eat, we ingest dozens of different chemicals and nutrients we require to maintain regular bodily functions. Once they are broken down, the body delivers them to where they are needed and then they work their magic on improving our overall physical health and stamina.

There are three main nutrients the body needs to keep everything running, as it should. Protein, fat, and carbohydrates, known as macronutrients, provide the basis of every function the body maintains from mental function to heart health. When we learn how to balance these nutrients in our systems using the calories we eat, we give our bodies the power it needs to keep running whether it is an average or extra stressful day.

Here is a closer look at the macronutrients and the specialized roles they play.

Proteins

Protein is the first of the three macronutrients the body cannot function without.

Protein is a vital nutrient that is most commonly associated with building and repairing the muscles and makes up about 15% of the average human body. While proteins can come from other sources such as beans and nuts, most people get the majority of their daily protein by consuming meats and other animal products like milk and eggs. For vegans, vegetarians and anyone else who prefers to avoid eating animals and their by-products, there are a number of plant-based protein sources like hemp and soy.

Protein plays other critical roles in the body including:

- Boosting metabolic functions
- Enhancing the immune system for stronger defense against sickness and disease
- Provides satiety effects that make you feel full longer after eating

While protein is important to the body's performance, it is also important to consume a healthy amount of it during eating periods. Most physicians and nutritionists recommend planning 15 to 35% of your daily caloric intake be devoted to protein. This is just a general suggestion based on scientific studies. The proper protein consumption levels are determined by several factors of each person including sex, age, and current weight.

When planning your meals, try to focus on eating complete proteins which contain all nine amino acids the body cannot produce enough of on its own. These protein sources are also known as high quality or ideal proteins. They are the best option for adding protein to meals because with them you guarantee that your body is getting the most out of each bite when eating. Proteins that do not contain all of these amino acids are called complementary proteins and still provide more than enough of the vital nutrients the body needs, only in less effective doses.

High protein diets are encouraged with any Intermittent Fasting routine to keep the body strong and feeling full during non-eating periods. However, it is good to consider the potential health risks that come with it before you jump into any protein-based diet.

Some of the most common potential risks and complications include:

- Heightened risk of heart disease and other cardiac concerns
- Decreased kidney health and performance
- Increased cholesterol levels and blood pressure
- Unexpected headaches and migraines

Men and women can both benefit from taking or consuming protein supplements either in pill form or in shakes, but never forget that protein supplements are not meant to replace high protein foods in our diets. They are simply meant to help balance any protein deficiencies a person may be struggling with.

Fat & Calories

The second essential macronutrient is fat. Though we are often told to avoid fats in our diet when we're trying to lose weight, there are healthy fats that the body needs not only for energy, but also for:

- Delivering fatty acids the body needs but cannot produce on its own
- Assisting with vitamin absorption throughout the body
- Promoting fat burning processes in the body when eating healthy fats
- Maintaining active reproductive functions in women. This is important as fasting can cause complications with the female reproductive system (as we discussed in the last chapter)

Eating fats to help increase weight loss sounds like an oxymoron, but it's true that eating the right fats actually assists in the burning of stored fats when eaten in proper amounts. This is because not all fats are bad for our health. Take a look at the different fats we eat and how they affect the body.

- **Saturated fat:** These fats are bad for your health and should be avoided or only consumed in small portions. Saturated fats are most commonly associated with obesity and heart disease. Red meats, cooking oils and butter are all examples of saturated fats that we eat every day.

- **Monounsaturated fat:** This is one of the healthiest types of fat we consume and can be used to help with weight loss when eaten in the right amounts. These fats also help with strengthening cells and lowering cholesterol. Avocados and vegetable oils are common dietary choices for those looking to add more healthy fats to their diet.

- **Polyunsaturated fat:** Another healthy fat, polyunsaturated fats are credited with providing the fundamental fatty acids our body needs but doesn't produce on its own. These fats focus on aiding and fueling vital brain functions. They are recommended for those struggling with heart disease as they help to lower the body's bad cholesterol levels and improving cardiac health. Polyunsaturated fats come from seeds, nuts and proteins like salmon. While this is a healthy fat for the body, it is still recommended to be consumed in small portions.

- **Trans fat:** This is one of the most widely available and unhealthiest fats people can eat. Trans fats are processed fats that have undergone a transformation known as hydrogenation. Through hydrogenation, healthy fats are converted into solid fat products like margarine as a means of keeping them from going bad. The majority of processed foods and fried foods are high in trans fats and only increase the risk of heart disease and obesity when eaten. In the last twenty years or so, people have been taking notice of and speaking out against the use of trans fat in products available in supermarkets, especially products targeted at children. As a result, there are more trans-fat free foods than ever before.

Many people use calorie counting as a means of weight loss whether they take part in Intermittent Fasting or not. Being aware of not only how many calories we consume each day, but where those calories come from is a valuable skill that can make all the difference when it comes to amplifying the amount of weight someone can lose through fasting.

Carbohydrates

The third macronutrient essential for the human diet, carbohydrates affect our energy levels more than any other kind of macronutrient. Carbohydrates (or carbs) contain glucose which the body breaks down into fat and is burned as energy for every one of your major functions from your brain to your tissues and internal organs. Carbohydrates are also responsible for affecting blood sugar levels and are particularly critical to monitor for diabetics and others with blood sugar-related health concerns.

While they are critical for the body to run, as it should, there are several different types of carbs and it's important to focus your diet on the more productive carbs.

- **Starches:** Starches are also known as complex carbohydrates because they contain longer glucose chains than other carbs. Due to their composition, it takes the body longer to process them and if consumed correctly, they can be beneficial to digestive health and a valuable weight loss tool.

- **Sugars:** Known as simple carbs, sugars are broken up into two categories of single and double sugars. Single sugars (fructose and galactose) are made up of just one sugar molecule. Double sugars (lactose and maltose) are created when two sugar molecules link up and form one sugar strand. There are countless sources of sugar we eat daily from desserts to milk products. There are also some grains and vegetables that deliver high amounts of sugar into the body. Sugars are made mostly of glucose and therefore do not take very long to be processed in the body. They contribute to increased fat production and blood sugar-related health risks.

- **Oligosaccharides:** These carbohydrates are a combination of starches and sugars that falls into its own category of macronutrient. They occur when 3 to 10 simple sugar molecules link up to form a long chain similar to the composition of starch strands. They take longer to break down than simple sugars on their own and have a sweet taste to them. Common sources of oligosaccharides include jicama, leeks, and wheat.

- **Fiber:** The final type of carbohydrate, fiber is also one of the healthiest for those seeking to improve their digestive function and increase their weight loss. Fiber is made up of both soluble and insoluble strands that the body is unable to burn as an energy source. Therefore, those who follow high fiber diets find themselves feeling full longer as the body tries to break down the fiber before removing it from the body and enhancing colon health as it does.

When trying to figure how to add a healthy amount of carbohydrates to your diet without receiving any of the negative effects they can trigger, the most popular method is to avoid adding simple sugars to anything you eat and only consume whole grains that are high in fiber. Other pro tips include:

o Go for the fruits and vegetables when looking to add fiber to your diet. Fresh is always best but canned or frozen fruits and veggies are okay as long as they are free from added sugars.

o Always check labels when buying pre-made or packaged foods! Even health foods can contain an unhealthy amount of carbohydrates that can set you back from your weight loss goals or health benefits.

o Fill your kitchen with legumes. Not only do they provide a good source for healthy carbohydrates, but they also serve an effective protein source that's low in fat and high in a number of essential vitamins like iron and potassium.

o If you can't give up dairy completely, try to only consume low-fat or fat-free dairy products. They contain less lactose, a double sugar that many people have difficulty digesting. Dairy products, when consumed in monitored portions, can be good resources for protein and fundamental vitamins the body needs to stay healthy. It's all about staying aware of what you are eating and how much.

Finding the Right Dieting Fit for Your Fasting Routine

Now that you know what the body needs from the diet that's fueling it, let's take a look at the most recommended type of diet for Intermittent Fasting and why it works so well with the program.

A variety of studies have shown different results for how effective different consumption levels of macronutrients in the diet can be for people with different body types, particularly those who are overweight and relying on dieting to help them take those pounds off. Despite all of the research done on the subject, there is still no definitive answer as to how much of an individual's diet should be made up of the macronutrients.

There is, however, a recommended ratio that can be adjusted within a range to meet everyone's dietary goals. Using the data collected through studies on a range of people of different ages, genders, and body types over the course of two years, top nutritionists and dietitians agree that in order to stimulate and promote weight loss without threatening the body's overall health, the balance of macronutrients consumed through calories should be as follows:

- Protein: 10 to 35%
- Fat: 20 to 35%
- Carbohydrates: 45 to 65 %

As with which method of Intermittent Fasting is best for you, it is impossible to say without some level of trial and error as your body reacts and adjusts to dietary changes. The key is to give your body time to adapt to a new diet before giving up on or getting frustrated with it. Always remember to talk to your doctor before starting any kind of new diet, especially if you have existing diet-related health issues.

How Should You Be Eating When Intermittent Fasting

The type of diet recommended for those trying Intermittent Fasting is one that is high in protein and low in calories. Since fasting is already the act of reducing calorie consumption for spiritual or health benefits, a lower calorie diet will only serve to help boost your total weight loss when using fasting for this reason. A higher protein diet helps keep the body from feeling fatigued during periods without food. It also helps decrease the amount of unhealthy fats and carbohydrates consumed when proteins are planned to take up most of the body's calorie allowance during non-fasting periods.

The Keto diet and the Mediterranean diet are two of the most widely practiced high protein, low-calorie diets on today's health scene. We'll take a closer look at these in the coming chapters. The following recipe is the perfect quick dinner or larger meal of the day for those using the Mediterranean diet (although many times dinner is the lighter meal on this diet, it all depends on your calorie allowance for the day) while they are Intermittent Fasting.

Vegetarian Stuffed Portobellos with Quinoa

Prep Time: 5 to 10 minutes

Total Time: 30 to 35 minutes

Makes 4 servings

Ingredients for Mushrooms

4 large portobello mushrooms, cleaned and stems removed

1 to 2 tablespoons coconut oil (or chosen substitute)

2 tablespoons balsamic vinegar

1 tablespoon lime juice or juice of 1 medium to large lime

Ingredients for Filling

1 teaspoon coconut oil (or chosen substitute)

1 ¼ cup quinoa, cooked ahead of time

1 tablespoon coconut oil (or chosen substitute), melted or in liquid form

1 ½ cups sweet potatoes, diced

1 cup red or bell pepper (depending on preference), diced

1 cup red cabbage, chopped

½ cup black beans, cooked ahead of time

1 teaspoon ground cumin

1 teaspoon smoked paprika or chili powder

½ teaspoon salt, sea salt or unprocessed salt is best

Directions for Baking

- Preheat oven to 400 degrees Fahrenheit if using the oven and prep a cookie sheet for the mushrooms.

- Mix melted coconut oil or chosen substitute, lime juice, balsamic vinegar, ground cumin, paprika or chili powder (seasonings to taste) and salt.

- Brush mixture generously over each side of the mushrooms and set aside on a separate plate.

- Heat a large skillet over medium heat and add 1 tablespoon of coconut oil or chosen substitute.

- When the pan is hot, add diced sweet potatoes and red or bell pepper. Cover and cook for 3 to 5 minutes, until the mixture is slightly browned. Remove from heat and set aside.

- Add chopped red cabbage and the listed amounts of cumin, paprika or chili powder and salt. Cook uncovered for another 3 to 5 minutes or until vegetables are soft and lightly browned.

- Remove from heat and transfer contents to a mixing bowl. Set aside.

- Use the same pan to cook the mushrooms by sautéing them for one minute and then covering them to steam for an additional minute on each side. Lay them on the cookie sheet, top down.

- Add all of the remaining filling ingredients to the mixing bowl containing the vegetables and mix thoroughly.
- Spoon the mixture evenly onto each portobello cap. (Don't worry if some of the filling overflows onto the cookie sheet.)
- Place in the oven and bake for around 5 minutes. (Toppings should be warm and lightly browned.)
- Serve on its own or with a diet-friendly sauce immediately.

Directions for Grilling

- Start by heating the grill. Once hot, grill your vegetables before dicing or chopping as instructed.
- Brush mushrooms with the seasoning mixture (described in step three above) and set aside until you are ready to start grilling.
- Once everything is prepped and ready, combine quinoa, vegetables, and spices (all of the filling ingredients listed above) in a large mixing bowl and set aside.
- Grill each mushroom about 2 minutes on each side or until cooked through.

- Once the mushrooms are top-down and face up, spoon a healthy amount of the filling into each mushroom and close the grill's lid, if possible, to let everything heat through. (Follow the final cooking instructions above if you want to finish them in the oven.)
- Serve on its own or with a diet-friendly sauce immediately.

*Sweet potatoes can be substituted for butternut squash if preferred or looking to give the meal a new flavor.

*For those who don't like mushrooms, eggplant, or bell peppers also make another great base for this dish.

*Use leftover filling can be used as a topping for tacos or a salad with your next meal.

Pro Tip: Grill the vegetables before prepping them, even if you're cooking the mushrooms in the oven, for additional flavor!

Leftover stuffed mushrooms are delicious, especially if you are doing any kind of meal prep. These mushrooms will store in the refrigerator for three to five days, but it is not recommended for freezing. The best reheating method is in a 350-degree Fahrenheit oven for three to five minutes or until the food is heated through.

Identifying Your Body Type & Why It's Important with Intermittent Fasting

Dieting is the best way to improve your results when first trying fasting, no matter what method or technique you choose. Intermittent Fasting affects each person's body in a different fashion so it is impossible to say with any certainty which form of fasting will work best for you. However, it is easier to narrow down your options when you can identify your body type and learn about which Intermittent Fasting schedule has proven most effective for your physical shape.

It is important to remember while you're trying to identify your body type that the body type you use for health and fitness planning differs from the body type you would use for fashion or sizing purposes. However, if you do have a good idea of your body shape and size it can be used as a solid foundation for finding your fitness body type.

According to health and fitness experts, there are four main body types when it comes to fitness. They are connected to the organs that affect them are widely accepted as one of the best tools to use to find out which diets, exercise programs or Intermittent Fasting methods will help you see the highest results. For this purpose, body types are determined by where your largest fat stores are located which tells you which

- **Adrenal:** This is one of the most common body types when it comes to dieting, fitness, and Intermittent Fasting. Those with the adrenal body type see the majority of their fat stores build up in the core and around the face. These are typically the people who turn to food when they feel stressed. The adrenal body is always behaving as if it is in a high-stress situation and releases cortisol from the kidneys that make the body crave junk food or sweet and salty snacks.

- **Liver:** People with body types shaped by their liver function typically consume higher levels of alcohol than others. It shows itself by focusing fat storage in the stomach to create a "beer belly" effect. High protein diets are not recommended for people with this body type because the liver is not functioning as it should, and increased protein consumption may only incite further issues.

- **Thyroid:** This body type stores their fat all across the body to collect not only in the core but the arms, legs and back areas as well. Other signs of thyroid imbalance can appear as thinning, more delicate hair, extensive hair loss or loose skin around the face. People with this body type often suffer from intense fatigue which they haven't yet been able to get rid of. The reason for this is usually a lack of vital nutrients in the body and can be fixed by taking a daily multivitamin.

- **Ovarian:** Women with the ovarian body type will store most their fat just below the belly button, as well as, in the hips and thighs. They will have difficulties with their menstrual performance and most likely suffer from an estrogen or other hormone imbalance. Women with this body type also tend to suffer from calcium deficiencies which can be balanced with a daily calcium supplement, especially if she is on a diet that allows little or no dairy.

Now that you have a better understanding of the relationship between your body and the food you eat, you can use that knowledge to find the right diet, exercise routine, and Intermittent Fasting schedule to target your problem areas and get you on the path to health and happiness.

Chapter 4: Intermittent Fasting & the Mediterranean Diet

The Mediterranean diet is built around the belief that the more whole foods you consume, the happier and healthier you will be. It is also one of the most recommended diets by professional health experts and fellow Intermittent Fasting enthusiasts alike.

The recipes are simple and many of them are vegetable-based. This is an especially helpful diet for vegetarians and others who may need to reduce or eliminate their meat-based protein consumption. For those who do eat meat as a major part of their daily diet, don't worry! There are plenty of ways to enjoy meat as a part of the Mediterranean diet.

Keep reading for a closer look at the Mediterranean diet, how it works and how it helps with any of the Intermittent Fasting techniques.

What Is the Mediterranean Diet?

Through comprehensive studies done since the 1960s, scientists have noticed and proven that people living in the Mediterranean region of the world (Greece, Southern Italy, Spain, and Turkey) have longer lifespans and less chronic diseases than people living in the United States. They discovered that one of the main reasons for this is because of the vast difference in daily diet between the two populations.

The Mediterranean diet is centered not on *how* they eat, but *what* they eat on a daily basis. The North American diet is filled with processed products, fast food, and chemical preservatives, while people living around the Mediterranean Sea take advantage of their environment and design their meals around the fresh produce and proteins the region has to offer. The people of the Mediterranean also consume a much higher level of fruits and vegetables than Americans who typically have an animal protein or processed carbohydrate-based diet.

The beautiful thing about the Mediterranean diet is that it changes the way people think about what and how they eat instead of just providing a handful of allowable foods that restricts your ability to go out to eat with friends or treat yourself to something sweet after dinner.

The Mediterranean diet is popular among culinary buffs working on their personal health, beginners to dieting of any kind, and people who have struggled with sticking to diets in the past because of the restrictions they had to adhere to. This is because instead of being presented with a short list of flavorless foods you can only have unsatisfying portions of, this diet and the recipes designed to meet its nutritious plan are full of delicious ingredients inspired by the Mediterranean. The Mediterranean diet is intended to teach its followers how to celebrate food and enjoy eating again with a new and healthy perspective. Each meal should be bursting with color from a variety of fresh ingredients and make you feel like you're not on a diet at all!

Most meals people eat on the Mediterranean diet are fruit or vegetable-based with healthy whole grains to further increase the nutrient levels of each dish. Whole grains take longer to process in the body than other grains and help you feel full for longer timespans after eating. This is an important factor to those choosing which diet is best for them while Intermittent Fasting, especially if they are planning to fast for more extending periods of time or fully fast on alternating days.

Salmon is one of the most common proteins featured in Mediterranean diet recipes because of its high level of healthy fats and wide variety of uses. Foods people should avoid on the Mediterranean diet include fatty red meats, processed foods of any kind but especially those high in sugar, and dairy products except for occasional small portions.

How Does the Mediterranean Diet Work?

For those who don't have a lot of dieting experience or have had difficulties dieting in the past, the Mediterranean diet sounds too good to be true. You aren't harshly limited on your brown rice or grain consumption, as long as they are whole grains. Fruits, which can be high in sugars, are one of the staples of this diet which makes it easier to satisfy cravings for sweet foods without reaching for a cookie or some ice cream.

At its core, the Mediterranean diet program is the definition of simplicity:

- Only consume whole grains and do so with every meal
- Center each dish around fruits or vegetables, depending on the type of meal
- Replace most protein from meat products with nuts and legumes
- Cut back on your salt intake by using herbs for flavor instead
- Enjoy some red wine, but in moderation

Many people following the Mediterranean diet not only start seeing weight loss quickly as their body adjusts to the diet but also start feeling better all over straight away. Increased energy levels, improved mood, and enhanced mental clarity are just some of the benefits reported in the first week or two of trying the Mediterranean diet.

The biggest change the Mediterranean diet makes for most people taking part is that it introduces fresher, more natural ingredients into their daily lives while eliminating the pre-made and processed ingredients Americans tend to rely on.

Here is an example of an easy and delicious Mediterranean diet recipe for beginners or experienced cooks and dieters.

Patsavouropita (Herby Greek Cheese Tart)

Prep Time: 5 to 10 minutes

Total Time: 35 to 40 minutes

Makes 8 servings

Ingredients

6 sheets of phyllo dough

7 ounces feta cheese, crumbled

¼ parmesan cheese, grated

2 medium or large eggs

2 tablespoons Greek yogurt, plain

½ fresh mint, chopped

¼ teaspoon nutmeg

Pepper to taste

Olive oil

Directions

- Preheat oven to 350 degrees Fahrenheit.
- Spread out phyllo dough on a clean counter or cutting board and lightly brush with olive oil.
- Crease phyllo sheets gently until they resemble an open drape or curtain. Repeat these steps with each

sheet of phyllo and use them to line the bottom of a large baking dish.

- Place in the preheated oven and let bake for five minutes.
- Mix cheeses, eggs, yogurt, mint, and spices to a large mixing bowl with 1 tablespoon of olive oil and combine until the ingredients are evenly distributed.
- Pour the cheese mixture over the pre-baked phyllo dough.
- Return baking dish to oven and bake until the top is a light golden brown (about 30 minutes).
- Serve immediately and enjoy!

Pro Tip: Sprinkling some additional feta or a light drizzle of olive oil over the top of the filling mixture before the second bake adds even more flavor to the dish. However, it is important to remember that all extra ingredients ad calories to the meal, so take this into account if following a strict calorie consumption plan.

What Are the Health Benefits of the Mediterranean Diet?

Arguably, the most notable health benefit of the Mediterranean diet is that it changes the way we think of dieting by helping people build a healthy relationship with food. It isn't just a temporary diet program to meet a weight loss goal. Instead, it actually inspires significant lifestyle changes with its available knowledge about how what the body eats affects our overall health. This is why nearly everyone who embraces the Mediterranean eating style sees more weight loss than with any other diet they've tried.

The Mediterranean diet is often praised for its ability to help followers with improving their heart health as well as helping them lose weight. The foods encouraged as part of the Mediterranean diet include higher levels of Omega-3s and monounsaturated fats, both of which help with reducing cholesterol and improving the heart's performance.

Other medical issues the Mediterranean diet has shown proof of helping counteract or control include:

- Diabetes
- Parkinson's Disease
- Alzheimer's Disease

- Digestive complications
- Chronic stress, anxiety, and emotional instability

Age-fighting effects have also been seen with the Mediterranean diet thanks to the higher levels of monounsaturated fats included in the program's daily recommended meal plan.

The Mediterranean diet program has also been with not only helping reduce the risk of developing cancer but for fighting existing cancer cells in the body. This is especially good for those facing an increased risk of cancers related to the digestive system like colon and bowel cancer. A major factor for taking full advantage of this health benefit is by replacing your cooking oils and butter with natural olive oils, the positive effects of which are widely studied and published in health and medical circles.

One aspect of the Mediterranean diet that people cannot stop praising is the fact that small amounts of red wine are not only allowed but encouraged for the health benefits contained in the drink. The recommended serving per day, however, is just 5 ounces for women and 10 ounces for men, as their bodies do not react as intensely to the sugars in the wine. This is great for people with active social lives or dine out with any frequency.

Are There Any Health or Dietary Risks with This Diet?

While there are many exciting health benefits provided by the Mediterranean diet, it is not always the best food program for individuals. There are not a lot of health risks associated with this diet, but it's important to understand issues that can develop, especially if you know you have a history of or already have a daily battle with their symptoms.

One of the dangers with the Mediterranean diet program is that so many people see the weight start to come off just by changing what they are consuming and let their physical activity decrease. While the fats contained in the Mediterranean diet are healthy for the body, they are still fats and can go from being a health benefit to a health risk if not burned from the body through regular exercise. This is something to watch as you get comfortable with the diet, especially those with a history of heart disease.

Those who struggle with a protein deficiency may find themselves needing to supplement the diet with protein powders or other means of getting protein into the body without adding a significant number of calories. If you have a history of this issue but don't want to take anything to supplement your diet, a more natural means of fighting low protein levels is to focus on vegetables and lean meats that fit within the Mediterranean diet and also contain higher amounts of protein than other food choices.

How Does the Mediterranean Diet Work with Intermittent Fasting?

Intermittent Fasting and the Mediterranean diet work hand in hand when it comes to improving overall health while increasing weight loss. Many dietitians and medical professionals recommend this diet for those looking to change their eating habits when starting an Intermittent Fasting plan.

Fasting is a major part of Mediterranean culture thanks to the prominence of Catholicism and Eastern Orthodox Christianity throughout the region. These versions of Christianity require practitioners to fast for spiritual reasons and as a show of devotion to their beliefs. The specific fasting rules for these Christian denominations vary with the Eastern Orthodox practice being the most restrictive and continuously observed (roughly 200 days each year):

- o Those who fast on Wednesdays and Fridays often embrace a vegan diet to get their allowed, but severely limited, calories as they can't have any animal protein or by-products (with the exception of organic honey), no alcohol (small amounts of red wine are encouraged on non-fasting days with the Mediterranean diet), and no olive oil.

- o Others embrace a fasting routine similar to the 16/8 method of Intermittent Fasting (covered in Chapter 6) where they skip breakfast each day and only consume two smaller meals later in the day.

- o The most devout and dedicated Eastern Orthodox fasters follow a fasting schedule similar to the Alternate Days Intermittent Fasting plan (also covered in Chapter 6). Their fasting periods last for 20 to 24 hours every other day and during these windows, they are not allowed to consume any calories from food and are encouraged to avoid calories from liquids or other sources.

The Mediterranean diet works particularly well for Intermittent Fasting practitioners that rely on calorie reduction and control to achieve their fasting goals. Even though their food consumption is still at the mercy of a minimized level of calories, the types of food involved in the Mediterranean diet are typically low calorie and are filled with good fats and nutrients that boost the performance of essential bodily functions.

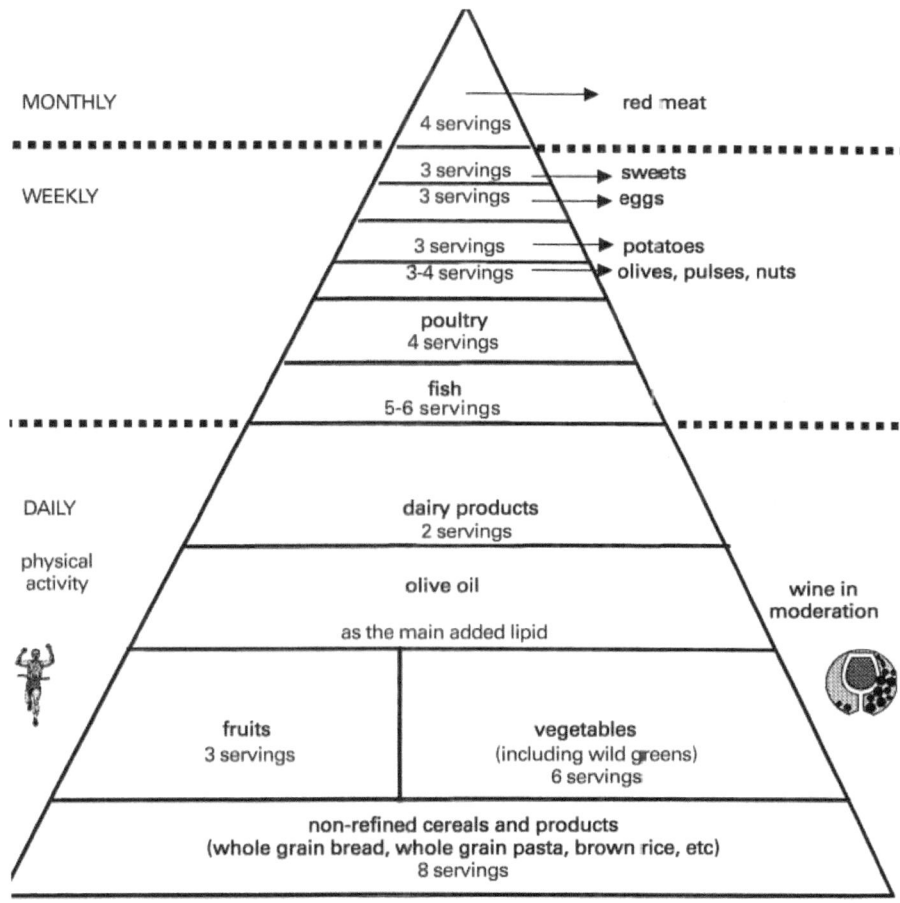

MONTHLY   red meat
4 servings

WEEKLY
3 servings — sweets
3 servings — eggs

3 servings → potatoes
3-4 servings → olives, pulses, nuts

poultry
4 servings

fish
5-6 servings

DAILY

physical
activity

dairy products
2 servings

olive oil

as the main added lipid

wine in
moderation

fruits
3 servings

vegetables
(including wild greens)
6 servings

non-refined cereals and products
(whole grain bread, whole grain pasta, brown rice, etc)
8 servings

One serving equals approximately one half of the portions as defined in the Greek market regulations

Also remember to:
- drink plenty of water
- avoid salt and replace it with herbs (e.g. oregano, basil, thyme, etc)

This chart shows a bit of a clearer view of what the Mediterranean diet should contain over the course of a month.

Many Mediterranean meals are also high in fiber due to the increased amount of fruits and vegetables many coming from traditional Western eating habits are not accustomed to. As we discussed in the previous chapter, fiber takes longer for the body to break down and helps you feel fuller for longer when eaten in appropriate amounts.

First popularized in a book by Michael Mosley, one of the most widely practiced methods of Intermittent Fasting is the 5:2 plan (which we will discuss in further detail later). The New 5:2 Diet is Mosley's recommended Intermittent Fasting program. His book of the same name combines the Mediterranean diet with a fasting schedule where followers eat normally five days a week and reduce their calorie consumption to around 25% of their normal daily intake for two non-consecutive days.

This is one of the most recommended schedules for women trying Intermittent Fasting because it helps prevent potentially dangerous hormone imbalances women may face when fasting for long periods of time.

Despite all of the evidence in favor of the Mediterranean diet being used to promote the effectiveness of Intermittent Fasting, there are those who believe that it may not be the best diet to use when fasting for a variety of reasons, including:

- Some people jump into the Mediterranean diet expecting dramatic results, but not taking into account the different life variables that can affect the diet's effectiveness such as age, body type, gender and health history.
- The increased whole grain consumption can affect blood sugar levels in those suffering from or sensitive to diabetic risks.
- Some people find the diet's guidelines to vague and loose for those using the Mediterranean diet as a means of weight loss. Inexperienced dieters and fasters can become confused about how much to eat and what kind of food they should be consuming and how much olive oil is too much each day.

Many of these concerns can be dismissed with the appropriate amount of knowledge about your relationship with food, how your body reacts to fasting, and what your body needs to function properly even through non-eating periods.

It is also important to remember when considering whether the Mediterranean diet is right for you that this diet program isn't intended to be used a quick fix for weight loss or as a temporary meal plan. The Mediterranean diet is meant to be treated as a way of adjusting your diet long-term for lifelong health and wellness.

There is no limit of information available about the Mediterranean diet and how it can help with Intermittent Fasting goals, so feel free to seek out more answers if you still have any questions or concerns. Always talk to your doctor before starting a new diet program, especially if you have pre-existing health concerns as they may affect not only the diet's effectiveness but also increase the risk of negative side effects.

Chapter 5: Intermittent Fasting & the Keto Diet

The Keto diet is another of the most popular diets recommended by those who've tried it while Intermittent Fasting to boost their weight loss and health benefits. Unlike the Mediterranean diet, which revolves around plant-based meals and protein sources, this diet works best for those who not only want to lose weight but also want to focus on their protein intake throughout Intermittent Fasting.

Here is a closer look at the Keto diet, the science behind it and how it can be used to increase the health benefits of Intermittent Fasting.

What Is the Keto Diet?

The Keto (or ketogenic) diet is built around an intensely limited carbohydrate intake and high-fat consumption eating pattern. It is a great diet for those who have seen success with low carb diets or the Atkins diet in the past. It is also recommended for Intermittent Fasting participants who suffer from protein deficiencies as the foundation of ketogenic diets is a dramatically increased protein intake.

When not in ketosis, the body uses stored and newly consumed glucose as an energy source for the mind, internal organs, and muscles. The main purpose of the Keto diet is to help the dieter abandon glucose as the main fuel source and focus instead on an increased production of ketones which the body can use as a healthier and more effective fuel source, especially when it comes to improving mental and cognitive functions.

We typically get the sugars we need for glucose production from carbohydrates and processed foods. When you start a ketogenic diet, you are encouraged to base your diet on natural food choices and nearly eliminate your carb consumption. Without the tools it needs for glucose production, the body needs to find another source of energy to continue performing all of its vital tasks. Basically, the Keto diet is the process of reducing your carbohydrate consumption and replacing those calories with fat so that your body enters a state of ketosis which burns fat and inspires increased ketone production in the liver to fuel the brain.

There are several different paths Keto dieters can take when they start their meal planning:

- **Standard:** The Standard Ketogenic Diet recommends dieters use a ratio of 75% fat consumption, 20% protein with a mere 5% of their daily calorie intake coming from carbs.

- **Targeted:** With this version of the Keto diet, dieters follow a high protein, low-carb diet of their choosing each day but are encouraged to increase their carbohydrate consumption around workout sessions. This version of the Keto diet is only recommended for those who are focused on physical exercise and professional athletes.

- **Cyclical:** The Cyclical Ketogenic Diet doesn't use a ratio for daily calorie consumption, but rather offers a schedule for how to stay in ketosis each week. With this version of the Keto diet, dieters use five days out of the week for ketogenic eating and two non-consecutive days for high-carb consumption, known as refeeding periods. This diet isn't recommended for those also following an Intermittent Fasting schedule as it can intensify and prolong the negative side effects of a ketogenic diet if not used properly.

- **Protein-Driven:** This version of the diet is almost identical to the Standard Ketogenic Diet but with an increased protein percentage in the base ratio. The adjusted ratio for those who want a higher protein intake is 60% fat, 35% protein, and 5% carbs.

Deciding which one of these options is right for you when stating the Keto diet is a matter of your body type and unique health goals. The Cyclical and Targeted Keto diets are mostly used by athletes and professional bodybuilders and are not recommended for use with any kind of Intermittent Fasting routine. Standard and Protein-Driven Keto diets are typically the best place to start for beginners and those who are adjusting from a high carbohydrate diet. These diets also have the most recorded research and study results of any kind of ketogenic diet, so those with questions and concerns can find all of the information they need before starting their chosen Keto diet method.

To give you some idea of how an average protein potion will look, here is a good beginner recipe that can be used for both daily lunches or lighter dinners on the Keto diet. These mini meatloaves also make great snacks for dieters who need a protein or energy boost between meals.

Marvelous Mini Meatloafs

Prep Time: 5 to 10 minutes

Total Time: 25 to 30 minutes

Makes 11 servings

Ingredients

1 lb ground beef

1 large egg

1 cup white or yellow onion, finely chopped

1 cup pork panko or chosen breadcrumbs substitute

¼ teaspoon onion powder

¼ teaspoon garlic powder

¼ teaspoon Italian seasoning blend

Salt and pepper to taste

Ketchup (organic or sugar-free is best)

Directions

- Preheat oven to 350 degrees Fahrenheit and grease your mini muffin pan. Set aside.
- Add beef, onion, pork panko, seasonings, egg, and salt and pepper to taste to a large mixing bowl and

combine by kneading until the ingredients are evenly distributed throughout the mixture.

- Take small amounts of the meat mixture (about ¼ cup portions), roll into a ball and then flatten slightly before placing in the greased muffin tin.
- Repeat until all of the mixture is used. The recipe should yield 11 total servings.
- Top each mini meatloaf with a dollop of ketchup and put in the oven.
- Bake for about 15 minutes or until fully cooked and lightly browned on top.
- Serve immediately and enjoy!

Pro Tip: To get the most out of this recipe, try to only use organic and whole ingredients. This includes picking up some grass-fed ground beef and organic ketchup or making your own ketchup from wholesome ingredients.

What Is Ketosis & How Does It Affect Your Body?

Ketosis happens when the body reaches a level where it is fueled almost entirely by consumed fat. When the body enters ketosis, a natural metabolic stage, it produces burns higher levels of stored fat and produces an increased number of small fuel molecules called ketones that improve the brain's performance when absorbed.

The following graph gives a visual of the steps the body must make to reach ketosis quickly.

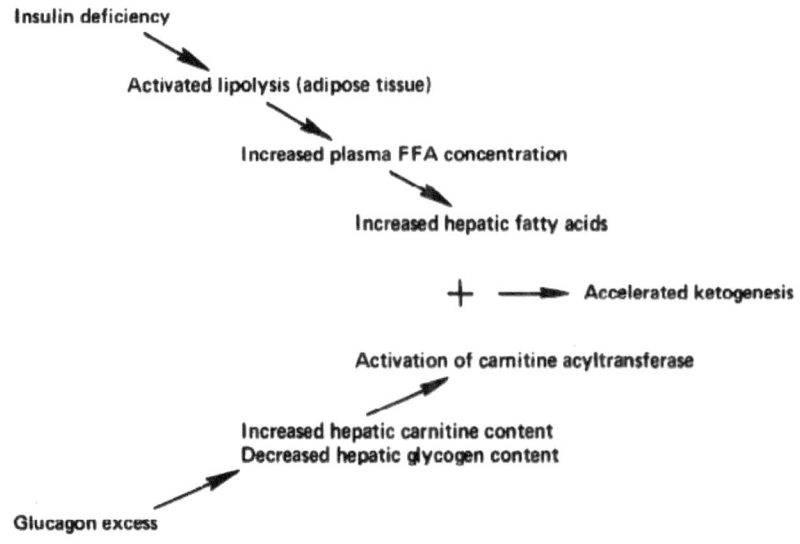

Biogenesis

Mitochondrial biogenesis is the essential function in the human body of creating new mitochondria from living tissue. Known as the "powerhouse of the cell," mitochondria are responsible for converting energy from the material in our cells and delivering it to where its needs via the bloodstream. The increased number of mitochondria produced when the body is in ketosis provides a number of health benefits. Most notably, a ketogenic diet has been proven to be useful in the treatment of rare mitochondrial disorders.

Glycogens

A ketogenic diet diminishes the body's normal amount of glycogen, a carbohydrate stored in the liver and the muscles. In order for the body to enter a true state of ketosis, the glycogen stores in the body need to be diminished. This happens when dieters are first adjusting to the severely limited carbohydrate levels consumed and is one of the main causes for the sudden drop in weight seen by new Keto diet converts.

While the initial weight loss can be a great motivator, it is important to know that the weight that comes off while the glycogen stores are being depleted is just water weight. Known as the Keto Flush, the drop of glycogen storage in the body can lead to intense dehydration in the first few weeks on a ketogenic diet.

The chart below compares test subjects on an average American diet (striped bar) to those starting a ketogenic diet (white bar) and their glycogen storage levels in the body. Over the course of six weeks on a Keto diet, tests show that the body stores less than half of the original glycogen levels it stored before the diet began.

In order to avoid this, it is critical to increase your water consumption, especially during fasting times if you are trying the Keto diet while Intermittent Fasting.

What Are the Health Benefits of the Keto Diet?

Weight loss is the most commonly experienced health benefit of any ketogenic diet and is arguably the main reason people choose to embrace them. However, there are a number of other health benefits people in ketosis can enjoy.

Recent studies completed over the last decade have revealed that Keto diets can be used to prevent and treat several neurological diseases including epilepsy and even slow the effects of Alzheimer's Disease in tested patients. It is one of the only popularized diets that has scientific backing of its effects on neurological enhancement in both animals and humans from children to retirement age.

Other health benefits of Keto diets include:

- **Acne:** This is particularly good news for teenage Keto dieters and adults who struggle with acne. Thanks to the lower levels of insulin production in the body, Keto diets often help improve skin tone and eliminate breakouts and blemishes.

- **Recovery from Mild to Severe Brain Injury:** This is one health benefit enjoyed by athletes who participate in high impact sports or activities. While human testing is still in its early stages, extensive animal tests have shown enhanced recovery from brain injuries include concussions and other physical deterioration.

- **Prevention and Treatment of Cancer:** Studies have proven that the Keto diet not only helps to prevent the development of certain cancers but assists with slowing tumor growth in the body for those already fighting cancer.

Are There Any Known Health Risks?

One of the most commonly reported negative side effects for those just starting a ketogenic diet is a phenomenon known as the Keto Flu. The Keto Flu usually happens in the first three to five days after dieting begins. Typically referred to as a period of just feeling generally sick, some of the symptoms include:

- Nausea and vomiting
- Physical weakness or lethargy
- Digestive complications or gastrointestinal issues
- Increased or chronic fatigue

While these effects can be intense depending on how the body reacts uniquely to the dietary change, the Keto Flu does not last more than a few days. Anyone experiencing these symptoms for extended periods of time or continuously should speak with their doctor about how to adjust the diet to meet their health needs or if a ketogenic diet is their best option.

The Keto diet isn't recommended for everyone because it can trigger or exacerbate existing health issues for certain people.

Diabetics, for example, should take extra care to monitor their blood sugar levels when partaking in a Keto diet. Ketogenic diets are known for severely limiting the body's insulin production. While this is one of its many celebrated health benefits, it can cause a problem for diabetics, especially if they are in the early days of trying the diet.

While many see improved muscle gain on the Keto diet, there are those who find themselves still losing weight but also losing muscle as they increase their fat consumption. One way of preventing this is to incorporate or increase muscle-focused and strength training exercises for non-fasting days.

How Does a Ketogenic Diet Work with Intermittent Fasting?

There are two main ways to get the body into a state of ketosis:

- **Dietary:** The dietary means of inducing ketosis involves taking on a high-fat, low-carb diet and sticking with it. Relying solely on a ketogenic diet to reach ketosis can take up to three weeks and can easily be lost with slip in diet such as extra carb consumption.

- **Fasting:** For those eager to get their body into ketosis, fasting provides a safe and effective means of doing so in just 48 hours. It is difficult to maintain ketosis when you only use fasting as a means of achieving it.

When used together, the Keto diet and the proper Intermittent Fasting technique can make all the difference in achieving your weight loss or other health goals. Intermittent Fasting can help the body reach ketosis while adopting a ketogenic diet helps the body maintain a state of ketosis through non-fasting periods.

If you've given your body an appropriate amount of time to adjust to the diet and are still feeling negative side effects, it may be a sign that a Keto diet is not for you. Feel free to seek out more information and talk to your personal physician about your options before and throughout any kind of dietary adjustment.

Like the Mediterranean diet, the Keto diet is not intended to be used on any kind of short-term health plan or as a means of rapid weight loss in a short period of time. Once the body comes out of ketosis, the beneficial effects of the Keto diet will disappear and the body will start storing fat as it did before the dieting began. For best results, the Keto diet is intended to be a long-term alteration to your daily eating habits to improve weight loss, maintain muscle strength and continuously enhance your overall health for a longer, more active life.

Chapter 6: Methods to Mastering Intermittent Fasting

Many people hear the word "fasting" and instantly make the connection with hunger and starvation. The truth is that they are very different concepts, one consciously practiced with a specific purpose in mind and the other an involuntary suffering.

Starving is the act of experiencing painful hunger, sickness, or death through forced periods without food typically caused by events that can't be controlled. This could be environmental factors such as famine, plague, or extended winter weather. It could also be caused by lack of food sources such as when someone is lost in a harsh climate or when a population surpasses its available food stores and production levels.

Fasting is the deliberate act of reducing calorie intake or refraining from eating for a set period of time. There are many reasons people choose to fast, but the two most popular motivations are for religious devotion and for taking advantage of the health benefits Intermittent Fasting has to offer.

Always wondered about Intermittent Fasting but weren't sure where to start? This chapter covers the technical workings of

Intermittent Fasting and breaks down the different fasting methods most used across the globe.

How Fasting Actually Works

At its very foundation, the human body has two main objectives: to store energy from food consumption as fat for later use and to burn fat as energy to be used as fuel for the internal organs, for sustaining vital body processes and other energy-related needs.

The first process is called De-Novo Lipogenesis, and it is most active during our peak eating times. It is the action of turning calories and sugar from the food we eat into fat stores that are deposited first in the liver before being spread throughout the body. Insulin is a critical player in keeping the body performing naturally and efficiently. When we are eating normally, the body's insulin levels rise in reaction to the newly ingested sugars and works to store them in the liver as fat cells. There is a limit to the amount of fat the liver can store at one time, however, so once the liver has reached its limit, the fat then travels to other storage areas such as the hips, thighs, and belly. The storage levels of the body are unlimited which is why we gain weight when we consume more calories than our body burns.

During times of fasting, our bodies activate a second essential process managed by the fluctuating levels of glucose in the bloodstream. When we aren't eating, the amount of insulin we produce falls, causing our blood glucose levels to fall as well. As soon as the glucose levels are low enough, the body kicks into high gear, pulling glucose from its fat stores until the sugars are all used up. When this happens, the body starts burning excess fat to maintain energy levels until we eat again.

Intermittent Fasting encourages those who follow the program to plan their fasting schedules around their current diet and lifestyle habits. This allows people to control when they fast so they can use Intermittent Fasting to balance these two processes and burn the most fat possible.

How You Should Eat When Intermittent Fasting

While many people exploring Intermittent Fasting already have a food plan, they are happy with, there are certain food options it's important to embrace or adjust your diet to in order to get the most out of your fasting. Keep the De-Novo Lipogenesis in mind when you are choosing your food for the times you don't fast. Think about how that sugar turns in to fat and spreads through your body. To reduce this action, avoid sugary foods, drinks, and excess carbohydrates.

One of the key elements to succeeding with Intermittent Fasting is supporting your fasting schedule with the right foods during non-fasting windows. Those dedicated to increasing their weight loss or muscle gain should focus on low calorie, high protein diets that boost the positive health effects of Intermittent Fasting. As discussed in previous chapters, Keto and Mediterranean diets are two of the most popular for people looking to change their eating habits. For those who aren't ready or have no interest in changing how they already eat, Intermittent Fasting success will depend mostly on sticking to your fasting schedule.

If you ask people who have been Intermittent Fasting for some time what they drink during their fasting periods they will tell you water, water, water. It is the easiest way to maintain the body's hydration levels without the risk of unwanted calories. Coffee and tea are also common choices. The trick to those that most people do not think about is that they have to be consumed without additional ingredients like creamers, milk, or sweeteners all of which contain calories that will interrupt the fat burning process initiated when fasting.

Another concern people have when first starting their Intermittent Fasting program is when or how they should eat during non-fasting periods. There is no one definitive answer to this question because each person will have unique responses to Intermittent Fasting and have to adapt their fasting schedules to eliminate these issues. However, experts do recommend that people fasting for shorter blocks of time have one or two larger meals when they aren't fasting and that those fasting for longer windows should have several smaller meals spread out over their eating time so as not to shock the body with sudden calorie intake.

The important thing to remember when you first start Intermittent Fasting is that just because one way works for other people while they fast, it does not mean that it will work for you. If you want to get the most out of your Intermittent Fasting routine, then it is crucial to conform your fasting schedule around your individual needs. This means it is critical to listen to your body and pay attention to how it changes and behaves in the first weeks of your fasting.

The Methods to Mastering Intermittent Fasting

There is so much information available regarding Intermittent Fasting that it can become overwhelming, particularly for those who have little to no previous experience with fasting. Talking with experienced Intermittent Fasting advocates can be just as frustrating as everyone has their own opinion of which fasting plan is the most beneficial.

The choice is often easier for women because there are certain Intermittent Fasting plans not recommended for the female body. This is because women's bodies react differently to fasting for longer periods of time than men's bodies do. These reactions can cause severe negative side effects if women don't properly balance their fasting schedules and pay attention to any symptom that may indicate a hormonal imbalance such as:

- Change in menstrual cycle timing or potency
- Increased fatigue of both the body and mind
- Unusual emotional instability or mood swings
- Change in skin tone or abnormal breakouts and blemishes

Remember that it is important to consult with your personal physician before initiating any kind of major dietary or fitness change. Your doctor can help you decide if Intermittent Fasting is right for your personal wellness and give more specific advice about fasting related to any existing health concerns you may have.

Let's take a closer look at some of the more widely practiced and studied forms of Intermittent Fasting so you can better decide for yourself how your fasting schedule should look.

Baby Steps: Start by Skipping a Meal

The easiest way to try Intermittent Fasting without diving right into a 24-hour fast is to simply skip a meal every day for a week. If that works, try another week to ensure your body has adapted to the change. This reduces your calorie consumption without a sudden adjust upsetting the body.

For example, start your fasting experience by skipping breakfast and only consuming two meals later in the day. This is a mild form of Intermittent Fasting that works by prolonging your non-eating window each day, if only by a few hours. It is recommended to give any new alteration to your Intermittent Fasting schedule at least two weeks to give the body time to adjust before making another step toward longer fasting periods or another reduction in calories. If after two weeks you feel primed and ready to make the next move on the path to Intermittent Fasting success, and then choose a fasting schedule that fits your needs and get going!

By starting here, first-time fasters and those simply curious about the trying the program will get a good idea of how their body is going to react to longer fasting windows without worrying about excess fatigue that can come with an abrupt switch to Intermittent Fasting.

Pick Your Window: The 16/8 Method

Once you know your body can function properly on one less meal a day, the next step is to choose when you are going to fast, how often and for how long. One of the most recommended methods for Intermittent Fasting is the 16/8 method.

Basically, people following this plan split each day into two periods: fasting and feeding. The most commonly practiced form of this method is 16 hours of fasting followed by 8 feeding hours where fasters consume a 50 to 75% of their former daily calorie intake. The easiest way to plan this is by continuing to skip breakfast by setting your feeding period to start at noon and end at 8 p.m. However, if you find this time table does not work for your schedule, such as those who need more energy later in the evening, feel free to change when your feeding period starts and ends. The time of day is not as important as the numbers of hours you dedicate to fasting and eating.

Although the fasting time is higher than recommended for females, women still find the 16/8 method beneficial because even though it is a longer period of time where they aren't eating, they are able to consistently consume a healthy number of calories every day. It is also the easiest plan to adjust to for Intermittent Fasting beginners and those who have trouble fasting for extended periods of time.

16/8 vs. 12/12 Intermittent Fasting Comparison (1 Month)			
Metric	16 Hour Fast	12 Hour Fast	Difference
Pounds Lost	9.8	12.1	-2.3
Fat Lost	2.7%	3.0%	-0.3%
Inches Lost	4.25	8	-3.75

The chart above shows a comparison of volunteers who tried two different time frames for one month of Intermittent Fasting. The findings show that those with more balanced eating and non-eating windows see more success over time. There are more intense forms of the 16/8 Intermittent Fasting method where participants fast for 18 hours and eat for six or fast for 20 hours and only eat for four hours. These plans are not recommended for women as the extensive fasting time and severe reduction of calories can damage hormonal functions.

The Ancient Warrior Approach

A lesser practiced and more intense form of the 16/8 diet, the Ancient Warrior method was created and developed by a former Israeli Special Forces member named Ori Hofmekler. The method is intended to help its followers improve their mental performance and burn excess fat from their bodies the way ancient warriors have throughout history.

Basically, the Ancient Warrior method involves eating little to nothing during the main hours of the day before consuming one large meal one to two hours before bed. This plan relies less on what you eat than it does on when you eat, but it is still important to choose the right foods when following the Ancient Warrior technique.

If you decide to try this fasting plan, use your restricted calorie count wisely and focus on low-calorie meals that are high in protein. This is one method that works well with the Keto diet.

Eat, Fast, Eat: The Alternate Day Method of Intermittent Fasting

At the other end of the spectrum, the Alternate Day fasting plan is practiced by those fully immersed into Intermittent Fasting and is typically saved for those fasting to promote spiritual health, the more experienced fasters or those looking for speedy results.

For those who choose this plan, the concept is simple: Avoid calorie consumption of any kind for 24-hour time frames, three or four non-consecutive days a week and eat normally the remaining days.

The Alternate Day Intermittent Fasting plan is ideal for those looking to lose weight and increase muscle mass because it targets the fat stores in the belly and hip areas without any additional physical exercise. Certain studies even suggest that this version of Intermittent Fasting works best for middle-aged people who are focused on not only losing weight but inches as well.

However, this is another method not recommended for women, especially those in their reproductive age. For those who are interested in only fasting on alternating days, the schedule can be amended so that instead of no calorie consumption at all while fasting, you would only consume 25 to 50% of your typical daily consumption on each non-fasting day. This is also a good way to gradually advance towards total fasting without experiencing adverse side effects and giving the body a chance to acclimate each time you reduce your caloric intake.

The 5:2 Plan: The Fasting Woman's Best Friend

As we've discussed, fasting for health benefits can be a complicated and confusing subject for women. There are so many factors and concerns involved with Intermittent Fasting that it can feel like an impossible challenge. The good news is that using the vast amount of research and expert opinions available, we have already determined the most highly recognized Intermittent Fasting option for women.

The 5:2 fasting schedule is essentially a modified version of the Alternate Day method, but instead of eliminating calorie intake, you would only consume a reduced number of calories. Most health experts recommend that people on the 5:2 plan restrict their food consumption on fasting days to just 500 to 600 total calories. This method also differs from the Alternate Day method. People following this plan only fast for two non-consecutive days each week and eat normally the rest of the week.

The 5:2 Plan works best for those as concerned about *what* they are eating as they are *when* they eat. This method encourages its followers to embrace a low calorie, high protein diet that will help them reap all of the benefits of Intermittent Fasting and achieve their health goals without having to completely abandon calorie consumption for any length of time. This keeps the body from entering survival mode and storing increased levels of fat in preparation for the next extended fasting period, canceling all of the weight loss benefits Intermittent Fasting has to offer.

Those hesitant about the health risks of Intermittent Fasting will also be interested to know that the 5:2 Plan also has the most scientific research and data supporting it, especially with regards to women's health. There is no shortage of data available or people who want to advise first-time fasters out there, so feel free to take vantage of all the resources you can find!

Why Is the 5:2 Plan the Best Intermittent Fasting Choice for Women?

Women have a tougher time finding an Intermittent Fasting schedule that works for them without the risk of hormone imbalance. While it is different for every woman, these imbalances can appear quickly and lead to greater complications as many of them are directly linked to the body's metabolic functions.

The 5:2 Plan is most recommended for women, particularly those who are planning to become pregnant or are interested in having children because there is never a length of time where you aren't eating that is long enough to affect the body's estrogen and other hormone levels in any significant way. This means that women who have failed to continue with a more demanding fasting schedule or have previously struggled with hormone imbalances while fasting has a new means of Intermittent Fasting that will not have the same negative side effects.

What Kind of Meals Should I Plan for Fasting Days on the 5:2 Plan?

With only 500 to 600 calories to consume, it is crucial to use them sensibly. Focus on making healthy food choices. Fill your refrigerator with lean meats and fresh vegetables. Avoid processed foods and stay away from refined sugars. Watch the calorie count of anything you drink during your fasting times to ensure you always have an accurate idea of how many calories you're ingesting and where they are coming from.

These suggestions are especially helpful for those planning on consuming their daily calorie allowance on fasting days as one large meal instead of spreading their calories out over their eating window.

If splitting the calorie count into two meals, have a smaller first meal and save your larger calorie consumption for your second meal so that your body has the additional calories your body needs to make it through to the next meal.

There are also those who choose to spread their 500 to 600 calorie consumption even thinner, relying on low-calorie snacks and several small meals throughout their fasting day. It is all a matter of preference and what works for your body specifically as you start your fasting routine.

This recipe is a good example of a light lunch or dinner option for those on the 5:2 Plan.

Indian Spiced Lentil & Carrot Soup

Prep Time: 10 minutes

Total Time: 30-40 minutes

Makes 4 servings

<u>Ingredients</u>

1 ¼ lb medium to large carrots, washed and grated (leaving the skin on is okay, peel if preferred)

¼ to ½ lb dried split red lentils, washed

4 cups vegetable stock or broth

½ cup fat-free milk

2 teaspoon whole cumin seeds, ground or powdered on preference (add to taste)

2 tablespoons olive oil

Chili flakes to taste

Fat-free plain yogurt and naan for serving

<u>Directions</u>

- Wash the dried lentils and set them aside.
- Wash the carrots and grate them. If you are not planning on blending your soup before serving it then it's important to grate them as finely as you can.

- Heat a medium or large saucepan over medium-high heat. If you are using whole cumin seeds, drop them in and toast them until they start to skip around the pan. Add a pinch or so of chili flakes to suit your tastes. Once toasted, remove half of the total seeds from the pan.
- Add olive oil, grated carrots, lentils, vegetable stock, and fat-free milk to the mixture and bring to boil.
- Reduce heat until simmering and continue to cook until the lentils are soft (about 15 minutes).
- Serve soup with a spoonful of yogurt and a piece of warm naan (or a low-calorie bread of your choice).

Pro Tip: If you want a smoother texture for your soup, transfer to a blender or a food processor and blend until silky. An immersion or stick blender will also work if you do not want the extra dishes.

This recipe is low in calories and high in protein making it ideal for anyone taking part in Intermittent Fasting, but especially for those following diets that focus on low calorie, high protein meal choices.

Which One Fits Me: Choosing Your Intermittent Fasting Method

As you can imagine, there is no one answer and a lot to consider with regards to which Intermittent Fasting plan is best for you. Especially as women, it is best to do plenty of research and talk to your doctor before starting fasting if you have concerns.

Our recommendation for those at the beginning of their Intermittent Fasting journey is to start small with skipping breakfast for a week or two and adapt from there. Pay attention to any changes in your body and alter your plan to counteract them. For those looking for additional help or want to share their stories, there is a massive community of experienced Intermittent Fasting experts and fans online that are always ready with helpful tips and encouragement at any stage of fasting.

Think you're ready to get started? Read on for our 14-Day Beginner's Guide to Intermittent Fasting designed with women in mind.

Chapter 7: A Simple 14-Day Beginner's Guide to Intermittent Fasting

As we've discussed, there are so many ways both Intermittent Fasting and choosing a diet plan that supports it can be practiced and no one way works for everybody.

This is especially true for women who have to take their essential reproductive functions and hormone balances into consideration every step of the way, making any kind of fasting or dieting program a more complicated experience than men have to deal with. Since the 5:2 method of Intermittent Fasting (covered in the previous chapter) is most recommended for women, we will be focusing on that for the guide contained in this chapter.

The first two weeks of any dietary, exercise or health-related adjustments are the most critical in determining how your body will not only adapt to but come to benefit from them. The same is true for starting an Intermittent Fasting routine, especially if you will also be starting a new diet that promotes the health benefits of fasting.

Before you start fasting, make sure you know how many calories your body will be consuming on non-fasting days so that you know how many calories you will need to eat during reduced calorie fasting periods. It is also good to know which two days of the week you will be fasting. This helps with both meal planning and managing your diet around any social plans or work obligations you would not want to fast though. One good aspect of the 5:2 method is that once you become comfortable with following the plan on a regular basis, you don't have to fast for the same two days every week. You can alter the schedule if need be so that you are fasting on different days, as long as they are not consecutive.

Here is a helpful 14-Day Beginner's Guide to Intermittent Fasting that gives you a basic Intermittent Fasting schedule to follow, an idea of what to expect and some useful tips from experienced fasters.

Day One: A Fresh Start Towards a Healthy Lifestyle

Congratulations on starting your Intermittent Fasting routine! This is an exciting step on your journey toward health. Intermittent Fasting veterans and health experts alike recommend taking a progress picture of your physical form on your first day as a means of keeping a record of your progress and for motivation to show you how far you've come on stressful or discouraging days.

With the 5:2 method of Intermittent Fasting, you will be focused on reducing your calorie intake to just 25% of your average daily consumption instead of completely eliminating food on fasting days. For most people, this means cutting your calories back to just 500 or 600 for two non-consecutive days each week and eating as you would normally for the other five.

Fatigue, trouble concentrating, and hunger are common effects felt in the first days of any fasting program. For those finding it unbearable at times, it is important to note when you feel the most hungry or tired so that you can adjust how and when you eat your daily calorie allowance on both fasting and non-fasting days. Some people do well having one big meal on fasting days while others find the plan easier to stick to if they break their calorie consumption into several smaller portions spread throughout the day.

Tip: Drink some water when you start to feel hungry. Dehydration can be an issue in the early days of Intermittent Fasting and hunger pains are just one of the ways the body communicates thirst.

Remember the feeling of success that comes with completing your first day of fasting. It may seem like a small accomplishment, but in order to stay motivated when Intermittent fasting and dieting gets tough, it's important to celebrate each forward step you take throughout your health journey.

Days 2 & 3: Past the First Hurdle

You did it! You completed your first day of Intermittent Fasting, and you can go back to consuming the normal number of calories for your chosen diet. While it can be a relief to know that you are not as restricted as you were, it is still critical to your long-term fasting to make healthy food choices even if you are experiencing unusual levels of hunger.

Here is a good recipe for fasters at any level for a quick, filling and healthy dinner that won't disappoint!

Superbly Stuffed Bell Peppers

Prep Time: 10 to 15 minutes

Total Time: 45 to 50 minutes

Makes 6 servings

Ingredients

3 large bell peppers, color can be of your choosing

1 lb ground turkey

1 cup broth, vegetable or chicken

8 ounces or 1 can tomato sauce

1 cup brown rice, cooked

1 ¼ teaspoon garlic powder

¼ teaspoon onion powder

½ teaspoon basil, dried

1 teaspoon red pepper flakes

1 teaspoon ground cumin

¼ cup sharp cheddar, shredded

Directions

- Preheat oven to 400 degrees Fahrenheit.
- On the stovetop, heat a medium saucepan over medium-high heat and brown the turkey. Add garlic,

onion, cumin, basil, pepper flakes, and salt and pepper to taste.

- Once the meat is browned and spices are well mixed, add broth and tomato sauce to the pan. Stir to mix ingredients, reduce heat and let simmer for around 5 minutes or until heated through.

- In a large mixing bowl, combine cooked rice and meat mixture. Set aside.

- Cut each bell pepper in half lengthwise. Remove seeds and ribs from inside and place each one skin side down on a baking dish.

- Fill each bell pepper with a heaping portion of the meat and rice mixture. Pour any leftover liquid into the bottom of the pan before moving to the oven for extra flavor.

- Move peppers to oven and bake for 30 to 35 minutes or until peppers are soft.

- Remove the baking dish from the oven and top each pepper with shredded cheddar. Return to the oven for 5 minutes to let cheese melt or put under a broiler for 3 to 5 minutes to add some color.

- Serve warm on its own or with a vegetable side.

Day 4: Your Second Fasting Experience

This round of fasting should be easier now that you have some idea of what to expect from your first fasting day. Since you are still in your first week, it's possible that there is still a fair amount of digestive discomfort or fatigue as your body is just starting to adjust to the lower calorie intake.

Pay attention to how you are feeling physically, mentally, and emotionally as any noticeable pain or change in behavior may be triggered by your diet or fasting plan and need to be altered.

Days 5, 6, & 7: Stay in Tune with How Your Body Feels

Back to your usual calorie consumption again! You may find that you aren't as hungry this time as you were coming off of your first fasting day. It depends on how quickly your body embraces the new food levels.

Tip: Spend the extra non-fasting day this week to mentally prepare yourself for your next fast and another week of Intermittent Fasting.

Day 8: Barely Missing Those Extra Calories

This is the fasting window that most people report as being one of the most difficult steps. You know what to expect on your reduced calorie fasting days and you've survived your first week.

Even knowing all of this, your third fast may be the toughest one you face.

One reason for this is that this is the fasting day where the concept that this isn't a temporary weight loss fix you take part in for a couple of months to get ready for swimsuit season. It's a lifestyle change that enhances your quality of life, but also has no measurable end. You've survived your first week of fasting, but you have a lifetime more to go. This idea can become a little overwhelming, particularly for those struggling with hunger pangs and fatigue.

Tip: The best way to combat this is to get active. Distract your mind from dwelling on your discomfort and stay focused on why you're fasting in the first place. Let your motivation and your goals be your drive.

Days 9 & 10: Looking for Adjustments

Now that your body is getting used to the reduced calorie fasting windows, you should be able to better identify and take action against any negative or painful symptoms you may still be feeling.

Maintain your diet and try to incorporate some additional exercise into these two days if you can. It is a good idea to start testing your energy limits as your body adapts to dieting and fasting so that you add or reduce energy-focused recipes in your meal plans.

Tip: It is important to understand what your body is communicating to you and to come up with a plan, but don't make any changes yet. Your body hasn't had the proper amount of time to adjust at this point. Wait until the end of your second week and make your changes then.

Day 11: Fasting Like a Pro Now

As previously mentioned, this guide was designed for beginners who are just starting their Intermittent Fasting journey. Most experts agree that two weeks should be more than enough time to understand how your body is reacting to both your diet and Intermittent Fasting schedule when any changes are made.

This is your final fasting day in this 14-day period and your body should have no problems with being physically and mentally fatigued or prolonged digestive discomfort. These are signs that there may be something off balance in your diet or that the fasting schedule you've chosen is not right for your individual health needs.

Days 12, 13, & 14: The Next Steps

Most experts agree that two weeks should be more than enough time to understand how your body is reacting to both your diet and Intermittent Fasting schedule. At this point in your new fasting and diet program, then this is the time to make your changes. Do you need to increase your protein intake? Maybe you're ready to cut your calories further or try a more intense form of fasting.

If you are still facing negative side effects, think about what is causing them and how you can adjust your plan to counteract them. If any existing health problems have gotten worse or new symptoms are appearing, stop the program immediately and contact your physician. They will be able to tell you where the problems are and recommend how to fix them.

Looking for more food ideas? There are hundreds of recipes and community boards online dedicated to low calorie, high protein recipes or recipes for whatever diet you may be following. All of the recipes included in this book work with almost any diet and help boost the positive effects of Intermittent Fasting in your body.

While the guide is designed to be used from the first day of a new Intermittent Fasting routine, it is highly recommended that you spend the two weeks leading up to starting your fasting routine easing your body into the many changes it's about to face by starting your dietary changes before you start fasting. Basically, if you are going to be doing a ketogenic diet while Intermittent Fasting, cut your carbohydrates and increase your fat consumption two weeks before you start your fasting schedule. This not only gives your body time to adjust to the diet but also gives you time to make any changes related to food consumption and to know how to identify these symptoms.

Chapter 8: Sticking to the Schedule

Knowing the science and exploring the different methods are just two parts of preparing yourself for Intermittent Fasting. In order to fully comprehend what you will be doing and how you should be feeling, it is important to learn about the most common mistakes made while practicing Intermittent Fasting and get some inspiring advice to keep you steady and determined through your fasting periods.

Common Mistakes Made by Beginners & How to Avoid Them

Beginner failure and success stories are the most helpful and relatable tools anyone getting ready for their own Intermittent Fasting experience can take advantage of. Knowing how others have struggled or soared when they first started fasting will give you a better understanding of what to expect, how to prepare yourself beforehand and how to react should any unseen problems arise.

Fasting Before You're Ready

One mistake beginners are notorious for making is jumping into Intermittent Fasting before they truly know what they're signing up for. As we discussed in earlier chapters, many people have a dangerous misconception of what it means to fast. People who haven't done their homework have been known to just stop eating for a day or two and then find themselves consuming more calories than they would normally eat because they don't understand how their body is changing as they fast.

This is dangerous behavior for both the mind and body as it can incite a variety of physical health concerns and lea to the development of severe psychological eating disorders.

You've already taken a good step toward avoiding these issues by downloading our guide to Intermittent Fasting for women. Never be afraid to seek out more information on Intermittent Fasting before you start changing your eating habits and lifestyle. The more you know, the more likely your success with Intermittent Fasting becomes. Read all of the articles you can find, talk to as many people who fast as you can. Become an Intermittent Fasting expert in your own right before starting and never start fasting until you feel 100% comfortable with the concept in general and the technique you've chosen to use.

Giving Up Too Soon

Consistency is the ultimate factor that determines anyone's success with Intermittent Fasting. Most experienced fasters and Intermittent Fasting experts report that one of the most common mistakes people make when they first start fasting is that they don't give their bodies enough time to catch up with the initially reduced calorie consumption. Since there are so many functions and processes in the body that are connected to what, when and how much we eat, there is no way of telling exactly how long each person will take to adjust to their Intermittent Fasting schedule.

The main trick to overcoming the urge to quit when progress seems slow or non-existent is to make sure you've given yourself the proper amount of time. For those struggling with initial fatigue and hunger from lower calorie intake, the symptoms should start to fade within the first week. If they are consistent after two weeks of fasting, that is most likely a sign that the Intermittent Fasting method you've chosen is not working for your body type and needs to be adjusted.

Give each adjust one to two weeks before altering your fasting schedule again. It may seem like a pain, but it is an important step when you first start fasting. The good news is that once your body has found a fasting schedule that works for it, you can build a routine and just let your Intermittent Fasting schedule become second nature.

Stay Away from Mindless Snacking

Another detrimental mistake that beginners tend to make is binging during eating or feeding periods. It is a natural response to hunger to want to stuff ourselves when we know we can eat again. This is a dangerous habit to form because subconscious binge-eating is one of the most serious threats to controlling calorie consumption. When the urge to binge overtakes us, it is rare that we seek out healthy food. This is the time that first-time fasters are more likely to cave and break out the potato chips or ice cream. It not only threatens the fasting schedule, but it also has the potential to undermine any health-conscious diet a person may be striving to stick to.

One way to avoid the urge to binge when you're not fasting is to make sure that you are satisfying any cravings you have when you can eat. That doesn't mean going straight for the cookies, but rather finding a low-calorie treat that quenches your sweet tooth so that you are less likely to give in to that temptation when it comes knocking. The same goes for savory cravings. Don't deny them, just find a way to fulfill them that works with your Intermittent Fasting plan and diet.

Stay Hydrated & Stay Sharp

Whether you are fasting or not, it is critical to the basic bodily functions of every human being that we consume enough water to avoid dehydration. This is especially true during fasting periods when water cannot be pulled from any food eaten. One mistake people make with Intermittent Fasting is cutting back on consuming everything during their fasting windows, including how much water they drink.

The trouble with this is not only does it increase the risk of dehydration and the complications that come with it, but it also works against the body's primary functions when fasting and intensifies hunger pains. In the last few decades, many dietitians and health professionals have told us that often, the hunger pains we feel during periods without food are actually the body letting the brain know that it is thirsty and needs water. Low levels of water in the body can lead to organ failure, mental deterioration and other health concerns that can be avoided simply by monitoring your water consumption to ensure proper hydration, especially when practicing Intermittent Fasting.

Going Extreme Without Proper Preparation

There are many benefits to being in full fasting mode and eliminating all calorie intake during fasting periods, but there are also lots of health risks that could be triggered if the body is not able to adapt to a newly started Intermittent Fasting schedule. A common mistake beginners tend to make, particularly those impatient to see noticeable weight loss quickly, is to skip easing their bodies into fasting and going straight for only eating reduced severely calorie allowances on alternating days and rejecting all calorie consumption for the 24 hours in between.

It is important to remember that fasting is not the most effective choice for everyone who tries it. There will people who can't find a fasting schedule that works for them because their body is just not able to conform to the changes that would typically happen with Intermittent Fasting. In these cases, there is usually an existing medical issue that may be fighting the fasting process. People who are already at their recommended weight and don't have much excess fat to burn will also have difficulties seeing any results with Intermittent Fasting.

The easiest way to keep from having to deal with negative side effects is to move gradually from reducing the number of calories consumed on a daily basis for a few weeks to whatever form of fasting they find works best for them. Intermittent Fasting isn't a process that can be rushed and the more someone tries, the more likely they are to give up on fasting altogether as their frustration grows.

Don't Stop Looking Forward & Always Strive for Health

Like with any diet or exercise plan, there will be difficult days and there will be lapses. The key is to always brush off all negativity that tries to cloud your mind and make you doubt your mental fortitude. When you start to get disheartened or feel your willpower slipping, just take a deep breath, get active and remember that you are stronger than you think you are.

Here are some tips to helping you stay motivated when your Intermittent Fasting schedule gets tough.

Know Your Goals & Hold Them Close

The more certain you are of why you want to try Intermittent Fasting and what you hope to get out of it, the more powerful you make yourself against negative thoughts and feelings that can threaten your determination. It builds a mental defense that will keep out harmful or tempting thoughts and keep you excited about your fasting program when things start to distract you. Answer these questions:

- Why do I want to start Intermittent Fasting?
- What is my ultimate goal?
- What is my dream timeline for reaching this goal? Is it realistic?
- Is there a more effective program I can try first?

Once you are able to fully understand your own objectives and motivations, it becomes easier to stay focused on both an Intermittent Fasting schedule and the diet you're following to maximize your progress.

When you find yourself questioning whether or not you can stick to your Intermittent fasting schedule, call upon those goals and aspirations to remind yourself why you are challenging your body. Keep them at the front of your mind or find a visual means of reminding yourself that you are working toward something wonderful like a dream board or a meaningful item you can carry with you.

Never Starve Yourself

Fasting and starving are two completely different sensations, one full of health benefits and the other a dangerous effect that damages the mind and body. If you find yourself being overcome by hunger and fatigue while fasting, especially those fasting for longer periods, it is okay and even recommended that you eat or drink something containing just enough calories to give you the boost you need to make it through the day.

Starving yourself works against the key processes that make any of the Intermittent Fasting techniques effective. It is always better to just have a low-calorie snack or drink like a juice or smoothie to ease any discomfort and find a way to make up it later. Get on Pinterest and start a board of low calorie, high protein snack and drink recipes so that you always have a collection of healthy food choices to pull from when you need to.

Here is a good example of a fun to eat, delicious and healthy snack that is gluten-free and works with almost any diet plan, especially the Keto diet.

Oven Baked Zucchini Fries

Prep Time: 15 minutes

Total Time: 45 minutes

Makes 4 servings

Ingredients

2 medium to large zucchinis, unpeeled

1 large egg

1 cup parmesan cheese, grated & fresh if possible

1 teaspoon garlic powder

1 teaspoon onion powder

½ teaspoon ground paprika

Directions

- Pre-heat oven to 425 degrees Fahrenheit.
- Line two medium cookie sheets with foil or parchment.
- Slice both zucchini in half and then split each half into quarters. Each zucchini should yield 16 slices when you've finished cutting them.
- Crack the egg and beat lightly in a bowl or other small dish.

- Combine parmesan cheese and spices in a separate bowl and set next to the bowl containing your egg.
- Take each slice of zucchini and dip in the egg until coated, then in the spice and cheese mixture before laying it out on the cookie sheets, skin down.
- Repeat the process until each zucchini slice is covered and on the cookie sheets.
- Cook for 25 to 30 minutes or until crispy, flipping halfway through.
- Pull from oven and serve immediately!

Pro Tip: Make sure your zucchinis are completely dry before you dip them in the egg. If they contain any excess moisture, the egg, cheese, and spices will not stick to them. Dab them off with a paper towel after you cut them and again before you use the egg wash.

These are great on their own but can also be enjoyed with a low-calorie dipping sauce. Stay away from mayonnaise or cream-based condiments. Any sauces or dips that you can make at home are preferred because you can control how many calories go into them.

If you ever feel bad about having to break your fast, just remember that one easy way to balance everything out is to slightly increase physical activity during your fasting times if possible, to help burn any extra calories consumed.

Treat Yourself When You Reach Your Goals

This doesn't mean go out and buy a celebration cake or order a bunch of takeout, but it is important to acknowledge your successes when they come to motivate yourself with when you start to feel uninspired or hopeless. Some people go shopping for some new clothes to show off their progress or take a short road trip to explore the areas around their hometown. Is there a book you've been dying to read or a particular site you've been wanting to visit? Maybe you want to sleep in a little later on your next day off?

Anything you desire can be used as a motivational tool or reward when it comes to setting goals for your chosen Intermittent Fasting program. Using this reward technique can also finally help you get more active and energized about your weight loss or health goal achievements.

Don't forget to take progress pictures either to share with your social media followers or to keep for yourself for motivation. This gives you a visual timeline of success to appreciate whenever you make another huge step forward or need to remember where you started and how far you've come.

However, if something sweet is your favorite way to treat yourself, there are tons of recipes online for desserts and sweet snacks that work with low-calorie diets.

Here is a look at one of the most simple and delicious desserts ever designed. It is a gluten-free, low-calorie dish that fits into any version of the Paleo diet you may be researching or following.

Honey & Cinnamon Banana Dessert

Prep Time: 5 to 10 minutes

Total Time: 10 minutes

Makes 2 servings

Ingredients

1 large banana, ripe and peeled

4 tablespoons of lemon juice

2 teaspoons of honey, organic is best if available

1 tablespoon ground cinnamon

Directions

- Preheat the oven to 350 degrees Fahrenheit.
- Slice banana in half and lay each piece on a lined cookie sheet with the cut sides facing up.
- Brush each banana half with enough lemon juice to lightly coat the surface.
- Spread one teaspoon of honey on each half and dust with the ground cinnamon.
- Bake for 10 minutes, remove from oven and allow to them to cool just enough that you can handle them to slice into 1-inch pieces.
- Serve warm and enjoy!

Pro Tip: You can put on additional toppings such as dark chocolate chips or miniature marshmallows if you want to but remember that these ingredients add calories to the dish that may affect your caloric intake levels for the day.

When it comes down to it, you are your own best friend and worst enemy when it comes to working toward your health improvement goals. Your thoughts and attitude can turn against you and make you question whether all the effort you're putting into Intermittent fasting is worth it. When this happens, it is important to find a way to make those thoughts disappear that works for you.

Conclusion

We hope you enjoyed *Intermittent Fasting for Women* and thank you again for downloading our guide. As you move forward towards your best self, remember that there are no cures for fitness and weight loss struggles. Physical health is a lifelong trek that is constantly evolving and needing adjustment.

This guide was designed to provide you with valuable knowledge and tools you can use not only with Intermittent Fasting but also for every step you take along your path to a longer, more fulfilling life. Any diet or fitness program you attempt will come with its own unique challenges, but understanding your body, your mind, and how they work together to help you lose weight will give you the confidence to overcome them when they appear. Use the tools contained in this guide to adapt to any life changes, to conquer temptations, and to stay strong when you start to feel disheartened.

Once you have chosen an Intermittent Fasting method that works with your schedule and decided on a diet that meets your health needs, make sure that you set an appropriate time to start your plan. Fasting changes the way you process food, and those changes can affect the body in unexpected ways. Fatigue, for example, is one effect first-time fasters experience and have to amend before they return to work.

This is why it is important not to plan your first few fasting days before major events or critical work obligations. Take a weekend, or any time you know you'll have a few days off, to start fasting so you have time to see how your body reacts and adjust from there.

Remember that knowledge is the best defense you have against difficulties that arise with any weight loss endeavor. Hopefully, we have provided you with enough information to prepare you for your Intermittent Fasting journey, but never hesitate to seek out more information if you still have questions about the diets, Intermittent Fasting or its benefits. There are also countless Keto and Mediterranean Diet books and recipes available online if you like ones provided in the guide and can't wait to try more!

If you enjoyed our guide and want to help others benefit from it, we would love to hear any feedback or success stories you want to share with a review on Amazon. We wish you the best with all of your health and weight loss goals and hope that Intermittent Fasting is the right fit for you!

Description/Pitch Page

The Intermittent Fasting for Women was designed to introduce health enthusiasts of all levels to the simplicity and effectiveness of Intermittent Fasting, specifically with regards to women's health. Readers will finish the book confident in their knowledge of Intermittent Fasting, how it will work best for their specific health needs and ready to get started on the path to a lighter and healthier life.

Intermittent Fasting involves controlling the body's calorie intake by blocking out periods of time where no food is consumed. Some people choose fasting schedules where they fast for a set number of hours each day, while others eat normally most days and strictly limit or eliminate their food intake on alternate days. As with any diet or weight loss program, it is important to choose the right fasting method to meet the needs of a particular body shape or health goal, a process wherein readers will develop a deeper grasp of as they make their way through this helpful and informative guide.

With this book, readers will discover the origins of Intermittent Fasting and how it has become one of the most widely practiced weight loss trends in the United States. They will also learn about:

- The pros and cons of Intermittent Fasting
- How to determine if fasting is the right choice for their health needs
- The science behind how the body processes food and how this affects weight loss
- The unique benefits and risks women encounter when fasting
- How to pick a diet that works with their fasting plan and supports a wholesome lifestyle
- The importance of eating whole foods and the difference they make when dieting

In addition to providing a comprehensive knowledge of Intermittent Fasting and the proven science behind the program, this guide contains introductions and explanations of two effective diets that readers are recommended to try while fasting to help increase their weight loss. The Mediterranean Diet and the Keto Diet are two programs gaining in popularity across the globe, mainly for their easiness to adapt to and recognized success. Each one has its own focus and food choices, but they both work effortlessly alongside any fasting schedule to boost all dietary benefits and help followers maintain a healthy lifestyle.

Beginners and fitness professionals alike will benefit from the book's 14-Day Beginner's Guide to Intermittent Fasting.

Complete with recipes from both the Mediterranean and Keto diets, this guide will walk readers through the first steps of their Intermittent Fasting journey with helpful tips and ideas of what to expect at each stage. To ensure their success, readers will also find information on how to avoid common mistakes and issues women face with fasting programs and useful tips on how to stay on track when fasting and dieting become a struggle.

Intermittent Fasting for Women provides readers with valuable knowledge so they can finally meet their weight loss goals with the help of a specialized Intermittent Fasting plan and a diet that reinforces the positive aspects of it. This guide is the ultimate tool and trainer for those looking to start an improved lifestyle dedicated to health, happiness, and well-being.

www.ingramcontent.com/pod-product-compliance
Lightning Source LLC
Chambersburg PA
CBHW051349280526
45784CB00007B/2879